AVAILABLE FOR GOD

About the author

Ian Newberry comes from Larkhall in Scotland. With his French wife Françoise, he is engaged in a church-planting ministry in France, where he leads monthly prayer-seminars. His aim is to encourage Christians and churches to develop their prayer-life and to be mobilized in a movement of prayer for France and the whole world.

DEDICATION TO MUM AND DAD . . .

You are the only two people in the world who know me from birth – as a baby, then as a toddler, as a child, as a teenager, and finally as an adult.

When I was a child, you – and my grandparents too – had a powerful influence on my life. You taught me to 'walk and talk' with the Lord.

Through your example, you burned into my heart the desire to pray. The flame of prayer has increased as years have gone by. That flame was ignited when, as a child of five or six years of age, Mum would take me on her knee before I left for school, read a story from the 'wee' blue book with a story and a verse from the Bible, then pray. That's when it all began. Thanks, Mum!

Dad too contributed to kindling that flame of prayer in my heart. Remember, Dad, when I worked with you 'in the fish' in the early hours of the morning. Before we left home in the van for the Glasgow fish market, you would say quietly but firmly, 'Let's get on our knees, son, and say our prayers before we go!' That too is how it all began. Thanks, Dad!

At every stage in my life – as a child, as a teenager and as an adult, when you saw my zeal for the Lord expressed through praying at home, in the church and in our little 'prayer group', and again when I decided to join the ranks of Operation Mobilisation – you did everything in your power to stimulate and encourage my commitment to the Lord and to fan the flame of prayer in my heart.

You yourselves were available for God. You were also available for your children, Wilma, Kenneth and Ian! You allowed me to make myself available to serve the Lord in France for over 25 years!

That is the main reason why this book bears the title 'Available For God'.

I pray that, as the readers turn the pages of this book, God will ignite the flame of prayer in their heart – and that each in turn will become *available for God*!

AVAILABLE FOR GOD

A STUDY OF THE BIBLICAL TEACHING AND THE PRACTICE OF FASTING

Ian Newberry

Translated by Peter Coleman

Illustrations by
Eric Boyer
Christian Munier
Anne-Marie Jourdan

OM
publishing

A WORD OF THANKS TO . . .

The Translator

This book was originally written in French and published by Editions Biblos. Peter Coleman, a dear friend and co-worker here in France, responded positively when I suggested he translate my book into English. Peter not only translated this book, but made some very helpful suggestions for adapting the content so that readers may come to grips with the thrust of what the Bible teaches about fasting. Peter, thank you for your professional touch!

The Artist

The painting on the front cover was donated to Editions Biblos by Madame Tournier with the prayer that it might help the reader to come closer to God. Thank you, Madame Tournier, for enhancing the presentation of my book!

The Photographer

The photograph on the back cover was taken by Sylviane Larché during a seminar on prayer, August 1997, France, and it is printed here with permission of the person photographed. I thank them both for their contribution.

© 1996, Editions Biblios
Produced & printed in France

English Language Edition published 1998 by OM Publishing
OM Publishing is an imprint of Paternoster Publishing,
P.O. Box 300, Carlisle, CA3 0QS, England
http://www.paternoster-publishing.com

ISBN 1-85078-318-7

Typeset by WestKey Limited, Falmouth, Cornwall
Printed in Great Britain by Caledonian International Book Manufacturing Ltd, Glasgow

CONTENTS

FOREWORD

In this day and age, dealing with the subject of fasting is certainly not the way to become popular overnight! Some refuse to consider the subject because it does not sound like a quick route to 'self-fulfilment' – apparently the main goal of our age. Others shy away from it because they are prejudiced against it by the abuse of fasting that has occurred many times throughout history. For example, some have treated fasting as a meritorious work performed to atone for their sins and to earn their salvation, while others have seen it as a means to obtain God's favour, and even to oblige him to answer their prayers.

We are indebted to Ian Newberry, not only for rejecting these distortions of the biblical perspective, but also for underlining the importance of fasting in the Bible, and for pointing out its fundamental significance as a sign of our availability to God and for God.

On the one hand, the Bible clearly teaches that salvation is a free gift obtained once for all by the sacrifice of Jesus Christ. On the other, it insists on the vital importance of giving ourselves wholly to prayer and of disciplining ourselves so that we 'may . . . be kept in soul and mind and body in spotless integrity until the coming of our Lord Jesus Christ' (1 Th. 5:23; cf. 2 Pe. 3:14). In our affluent society, we badly need to remember the warning given by Jesus: 'Be on your guard – see to it that your minds are never clouded by dissipation or drunkenness or the worries of this life, or else that may catch you like the springing of a trap' (Lk. 21:34).

When the apostle Paul stated: 'I am my body's sternest master, for fear that when I have preached to others, I should myself be disqualified' (1 Co. 9:27), no doubt he included in his severe treatment of his body the fact that he had often done without meals (cf. 2 Co. 11:27). The disqualification he feared certainly included the lack of availability for listening to God and for carrying out 'all those good deeds which God has planned for us to do'.

While our fellow-Christians in Eastern Europe often still have to be content with only one meal a day, we in the West need to be reminded of the considerable benefits to health that accrue from fasting.* Above all, in an age when we are sometimes too busy to take time even for the essential things of life, we need to remember the main benefit of fasting: it enables us to be available to God and for God.

Alfred Kuen

* Laboratory experiences have demonstrated that rats obliged to fast once a week live 33% longer than the others!

PREFACE

The exemplary lives of men and women of prayer who have practised fasting and the impact they made on their generation motivated me to think about the subject of fasting and to study and practise it.

A Christian magazine asked me to write two articles, one on fasting individually and one on group fasting, with the title 'Available to God'. I first considered what the Bible says about fasting. Then I spoke to pastors, theologians and doctors, in order to gather still more information on the subject.

Little has been written in French about fasting whether by Catholic or Protestant authors. However, I was able to glean ideas and information from a few articles and pamphlets, and to derive much help from Catherine Gotte's thesis presented to the Free Evangelical Theological Seminary at Vaux-sur-Seine, Paris, and entitled 'Towards A Better Understanding of Fasting In Christian Spirituality'.

I had great pleasure ferreting out old books in big libraries in order to discover what had been written about fasting by the Church Fathers, the Reformers and other men of God who have kept 'the pattern of sound doctrine'. I would like to thank those responsible for the following libraries who allowed me to consult their books:

- The Palais Bourbon Library, Paris

- The Free Evangelical Seminary, Vaux-sur-Seine

- The Nogent-sur-Marne Bible Institute

- The Montélimar Médiathèque

- The Les Fontaines Library at Chantilly

- The Aiguebelle Abbey Library

- The Emmaus Bible Institute, Saint-Légier, Vevey, Switzerland

- The Church of Scotland College Library, Edinburgh, Scotland

Here is how this book was born: after wondering about certain questions, studying the Bible and interviewing various people, I wrote two articles on fasting and prayer for a Christian magazine, then composed a small manual for the participants in a seminar on fasting. I then pursued this study further and decided to turn it into a book for the general public.

This book is now in your hands because several friends have encouraged and advised me and have corrected my initial manuscript. I wish to thank them for their patience and for their suggestions and constructive criticisms.

A book written amidst the nitty-gritty of everyday life

I am involved in church-planting in the south of France. I was able to use odd moments in a busy life to read up my subject and put my thoughts into writing – not only in my study at home and in various libraries, but also sitting behind my Friday-morning bookstall in the market, travelling by bus and train, and even in my deckchair by the river Gardon or by the Mediterranean sea while on holiday!

How this book is set out

How should I present this material so that the reader can understand the gist of it? You will notice that priority has been given to the biblical teaching. Relatively little space has been devoted to historical, medical and therapeutic aspects.

Nonetheless it was thought useful to give – in two appendices – a brief overview of fasting throughout the history of the church and concise information about the way fasting is practised in the major world religions.

All quotations other than those from the Bible have been numbered. You will find references to the authors and titles at the end of the book.

Questions for further reflection

At the end of each chapter you will find questions to encourage you to undertake further reflection and study on this material and to put it into practice. I strongly encourage you to work through these questions using pencil and paper, either alone or in a group. This will help you to turn theory into practice!

My prayer for you

The author's prayer is that the reading of this book and especially the consideration of the passages from the Bible will enable you to gain a clear understanding of the meaning of fasting. May this study help you to take practical measures with a view to becoming available to God in the enjoyment of his presence!

Prayer: 'Lord, draw my heart to You, make me thirsty for your presence and for your Word, and may this experience remain a priority in my everyday life.'

Pierrelatte, 1997
Ian Newberry

ABBREVIATIONS

Old Testament

Genesis . . . . Ge
Exodus . . . . Ex
Leviticus . . . . . . Lev
Numbers . . . . Nu
Deuteronomy . . . . Dt
Judges . . . . Jdg
1/2 Samuel . . . . 1/2 Sam
1 Kings . . . . 1 Ki
1/2 Chronicles . . . 1/2 Ch
Ezra . . . . Ezr
Nehemiah . . . . . . Ne
Esther . . . . Est
Job . . . . Job
Psalms . . . . Ps
Isaiah . . . . Isa
Jeremiah . . . . Jer
Daniel . . . . Da
Joel . . . . Joel
Jonah . . . . Jnh
Zechariah . . . . . . Zec

New Testament

Matthew . . . . Mt
Mark . . . . Mk
Luke . . . . Lk
John . . . . Jn
Acts . . . . Ac
Romans . . . . Ro
1/2 Corinthians . . . 1/2 Co
Galatians . . . . Gal
Colossians . . . . . . Col
1 Thessalonians . . . 1 Th
1 Timothy . . . . . . 1 Ti
Hebrews . . . . Heb
James . . . . Jas
2 Peter . . . . 2 Pe
1 John . . . . 1 Jn

Apocrypha

1/2 Esdras . . . . . . 1/2 Esd

Unless otherwise stated,

– New Testament quotations are from The New Testament in Modern English by J.B. Phillips (1960);

– Old Testament quotations are from The Holy Bible, New International Version (1973, 1978, 1984).

CHAPTER 1   INTRODUCTION

1. The purpose of this book

2. The urgency of this teaching

3. Three testimonies:
    - The testimony of the church down through history
    - My personal testimony
    - The testimony of a particular church

4. Definitions and quotations

5. Questions for further reflection

Fasting is neither an end in itself nor even a means to an end; it is an expression of one's confidence in God, of one's availability to him, and of one's dependence on him as one seeks to meet with him.

1. The purpose of this book

I am glad that this book has come into your possession!

I am sure you have a burning desire to obtain a perfectly clear answer to the question: What does the Bible teach concerning fasting, individually and collectively?

I too asked myself this question. It led me to ask other questions:

Is fasting obligatory? What is the purpose of fasting? When should one fast? In what way and in what circumstances should one fast? How long should one fast? How should one prepare to fast? How should one terminate one's fast? Is fasting dangerous for one's health?

I hope that by the time you have finished reading this book you will have discovered a clear biblical answer to all these questions. I hope especially that you will have understood the fundamental meaning of fasting in Scripture and that you will have learned to practise fasting wisely and for biblical reasons.

Before going any further, I would like you to test your knowledge of the biblical teaching about fasting. On page 3, please put an X against what you think is the correct answer:

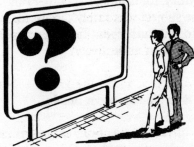

A LITTLE TEST OF WHAT YOU KNOW ABOUT FASTING

	RIGHT	WRONG	DON'T KNOW
1. In the Bible, fasting is mentioned 8 times; it is practised by 5 people in exceptional circumstances.			
2. In the Bible, the word 'fasting' can mean 'humbling oneself before God'.			
3. Jesus practised fasting, but he did not explain how or why one should fast.			
4. Isaiah 58 deals with right and wrong motives for fasting.			
5. Group fasting was often practised in the Old Testament, but never in the New Testament.			
6. In the Bible, fasting was always practised with a view to obtaining an answer to prayer.			
7. In Scripture, God himself speaks about fasting.			
8. The Bible refers to fasting more than seventy times.			

Much ado – followed by nothing

At certain times in history, people have talked a great deal about fasting – in the 4th century, for example. At other times – as at the present time – the subject was rarely discussed. If the Holy Spirit guides us into the truth about fasting, we will avoid falling into either of these extremes.

A. The purpose of this book is to illuminate our minds

For too long the subject of fasting has been shrouded in ignorance and silence. In the last forty years, I must have attended more than eight thousand meetings of one sort or another, but I have never heard teaching on fasting. Practically no book on fasting was published between 1861 and 1954, and even today few books dealing with fasting from a Christian standpoint are widely available.

Now, if you have completed the test on p. 3, you can look at the right answers which are found on p. 37.

B. **The purpose of this book is to encourage us to be more available to God**

The word 'available' also means 'free'. It implies freeing ourselves from all other constraints and obligations in order to concentrate completely on one particular task.

Sometimes people take a 'sabbatical' year off their usual work in order to be 'free' to study, to train – or to travel.

On my desk lies a big red diary. Each evening I prepare a list of things to do the following day. Then I arrange them according to their importance. Each day I note my number one priority: a task I absolutely must undertake that day – no matter how the day turns out, whatever interruptions may occur, or however I feel at the moment.

This morning, for example, I have a long list of things I must do: phone several people, prepare a Bible study, organize my next seminar, make some visits, purchase my train ticket . . .

However, for me the highest priority every day is to make myself available to God.

Every morning, I drive some distance out of town, park on a little country road bordered by vines and continue on foot. As I walk, I talk aloud to the Lord – just as I would to a friend. I am literally going for a walk in his company. However many tasks I must undertake every day, my first priority is to be available to God early each morning.

God desires that our heart, our spirit, and indeed our whole life be available to him. He wants to fill them with his presence, his power and his Word.

God desires not only to meet with us, but to do us good. He wants to listen to us. That is why he has given us this beautiful promise:

'The Lord is near to all who call upon him, to all who call on him in truth. He fulfils the desires of those who fear him; he hears their cry and saves them' (Ps. 145:18–19).

2. The urgency of this teaching

Should we speak about fasting?

People have often said to me: 'Ian, we would like you to speak to us about fasting – but please don't make a meal of it!'

I must admit that I hesitated a long time before taking up my pen to write this book. I was afraid of writing about this subject without having studied it sufficiently. I was afraid too of studying it without also knowing the joy of experiencing the presence of God while practising this discipline.

For a number of years, I have researched the subject of fasting and I have practised fasting for the following reasons:

The Bible speaks about it

More than seventy verses allude to fasting, and many examples of the practice are mentioned.

The Old Testament gives numerous examples of fasting practised both individually and collectively. These examples show that fasting is an outward sign of inward sorrow. The prophets Isaiah and Zechariah warn about right and wrong motivations for fasting (see Isa. 58 and Zec. 7).

In the New Testament, Jesus explains why and how we should fast (see Mt.6:16–18). The apostle Paul warns against the danger of going to extremes (see Col. 2:20–23). The purpose and practice of fasting in the local church are illustrated by the practice of the early Christians (see Ac. 13:3).

The giants of faith in the Bible have shown the way

We can learn an enormous amount by considering and imitating the great cloud of witnesses which includes Moses (Ex. 34:28), Samuel (1 Sam. 7:6), David (Ps. 69:10–21), Jonathan (1 Sam. 20:34), Jehoshaphat (2 Ch. 20:3), Ezra (Ezr. 10:6), Nehemiah (Ne. 1:4–10), Daniel (Da. 9:3), Esther (Est. 4:10–17), Elijah (2 Ki. 19:8), Joel (Joel 1:14), Zechariah (Zec. 8:18), and the people of Israel (Jdg. 8:26-28). In addition the annual day of fasting was an important date in the Hebrew calendar (Lev. 16:29).

To this long list, the New Testament adds Anna the prophetess (Lk. 2:37), John the Baptist and his disciples (Lk. 5:33), Jesus (Mt. 4:2), Paul (2 Co. 6:5), the elders at Antioch (Ac. 13:3), and the church at Lystra (Ac. 14:23).

The giants of faith down through the history of the church have left us an example

The history of the church reveals that fasting and prayer have often preceded times of revival. Try to obtain and read the biographies of men of prayer like . . .

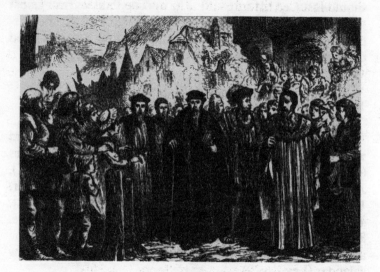

Calvin arriving at Geneva

. . . Tertullian, Origen, Jerome, Augustine, Martin Luther, Calvin, John Knox (a Scot on fire for God!), Jonathan Edwards, David Brainard, John and Charles Wesley, Charles G. Finney, D.L. Moody, Watchman Nee, Pastor Hsi of China, Hudson Taylor, George Verwer . . . *All of them practised prayer and fasting.*

The danger of falling into the trap of syncretism

Fasting is taught and practised not only in the Catholic Church and the Orthodox Church, but also in the major non-Christian religions like Hinduism, Buddhism and Islam, by notable religious figures like Confucius, Zoroaster, by various famous yogis of India, by great philosophers such as Plato, Socrates and Aristotle, and also by Hippocrates, the Greek physician commonly regarded as the father of medicine.

In my research, I was surprised to discover that fasting is taught and practised not only in the major non-Christian religions of the world, but also in some occult movements.

Syncretism is the attempt to combine in one system the characteristic ideas and practices of different philosophies and religions.

The resulting mixture of mystical ideas and ascetic practices leads to a quite different understanding of fasting from what the Bible teaches about it.

Certain Christians go from one extreme to another

Amongst Christians, one can meet two extremes: some practise fasting but not in a biblical way, while others know the biblical teaching but do not put it into practice.

Biblical fasting must not be confused with other kinds of fasting

For some, fasting is a way to experience a feeling of ecstasy. For others, it is a way of strengthening their will-power or of accomplishing a feat of asceticism. Fasting may also be practised to improve health and fitness. We will have little to say about those kinds of fasting.

There is *no* spiritual value whatever in practising fasting in an unbiblical way, in other words, *without* prayer (without humbling oneself, giving thanks, interceding for others . . .).

Fasting must spring from a personal conviction based on the Word of God.

The purpose of this study is not to enable you to become an expert at fasting, but rather to help you consider what the Bible teaches on the subject and to follow the Biblical pattern.

3. Three testimonies

The testimony of the church down through history

The teaching and practice of fasting in the church down through history can be summarized as 'Much ado – followed by nothing!'

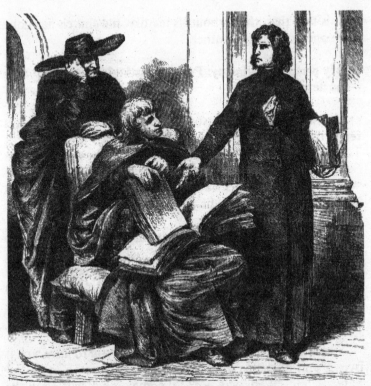

A group of intellectuals study the Holy Scriptures

For example, in the 3rd and 4th centuries, fasting was considered an important aspect of the Christian's discipline of his body. At other times little was said about fasting. This appears to be the case at present. After several inquiries, I realised that fasting is not much in vogue these days in Evangelical churches – though there are some exceptions, of course.

Why is fasting so rarely mentioned nowadays? What ideas does the word 'fasting' bring to your mind? Asceticism? Suffering? Fanaticism? Forcing oneself to do something against one's will?

11

It is true that, throughout its history, the church has gone from one extreme to another.

My personal testimony: Practise fasting? That's not for me – and never will be!

When the subject of fasting comes to mind, I will always remember the year I spent with Operation Mobilisation at Tours, in France. The whole team would be seated around a big table, ready to begin the meal. Then someone would ask: 'Where's Bob? What's he doing now?' Bob was our team leader. A man of prayer, he often went missing at mealtimes.

Every Friday evening, Bob went out on the streets to invite new people to an evangelistic event, but first he led his team in a time of fervent prayer. I can assure you, he contacted new people in the street and brought them to the 'coffee-bar' as easily as my grandmother could put stitches onto her knitting-needles!

'Good evening! We would like to invite you to have a chat over a cup of coffee in a friendly atmosphere . . . to a debate . . .' etc. 'Well, why not? I'll come along!' was often the reply. We accompanied our contacts to our coffee-bar (a 'converted' cellar), introduced them to the local Christians, and returned to the streets to fetch other 'fish' that Bob had 'caught' in the meantime. This went on for an hour or so. By now, our little coffee-bar was brimful with all sorts of people: students, hippies, tramps, young people, old couples, Africans, Asians – and even Scots – all sitting on the carpet, two to the square yard!

A little music, a few songs, two brief testimonies and a forceful ten-minute message were followed by discussion over a cup of coffee. Conversation continued into the early hours as people began to pass from darkness into light.

Dozens of people came to Christ in this way! What methods did you use? Tell us so we can try it in our church!

Here's my explanation: one man on his knees in prayer. Bob could pray his way around the world as easily as you can walk around a table! For him, prayer was as natural as breathing!

There were five fellows on our team, and we shared the same bedroom. Often, at 3 a.m., we caught sight of a silhouette crossing the room and climbing the ladder to the third-storey bunk-bed. Bob had just spent the first part of the night in prayer!

Not only was Bob's bed often empty, but his place at table too. His frequent absences at mealtimes intrigued me. Practise fasting? That's not for me – and never will be! My mother had spent nearly twenty years trying to get me to eat whatever was on the table so that I would become a healthy young man – she would be sick with anxiety if she learned that I was going without meals. No thanks, Bob, fasting's not for me and never will be!

The testimony of a particular church

In order to help solve a problem that had arisen in the church, one of the leaders proposed a day of prayer and fasting. Not everyone agreed with the proposal, and some were even quite opposed. What should we do? Some quoted the example of Hudson Taylor, the famous founder of the China Inland Mission: he used to practise fasting every time he encountered a major problem. Others quoted Isaiah 58 which criticizes the kind of fasting practised in Israel at that time.

13

After some talk about the danger of letting Jewish legalism and asceticism squeeze out the grace of God, we finally agreed to look for the answer in the Bible.

This is precisely what we want to do together now.

4. Definitions and quotations

Fast. To abstain from eating all or certain foods or meals, especially as a religious observance. An act or a period of fasting. *Collin's English Dictionary*

To understand the origin of the expression, we only have to think of the familiar term "breakfast" – which means just what it says: "breaking a fast". So fasting simply implies abstaining from food for a certain time.

What great times we have at table when the soup is steaming, the roast is in the oven, the ice cream is in the fridge and the coffee is beginning to percolate. 'We'll just give thanks and then dig in!' After all, we are hungry and we need food to give us energy.

Unfortunately the word fasting conjures up all sorts of fears. For some fasting is synonymous with suffering: it entails forcing oneself to go without food and losing weight. However, those fears disappear when we study the Scriptures and discover the meaning of fasting in the Bible.

Fasting defined by the Bible

It is important to allow the Bible itself to define fasting for us.

God himself asks the question: 'Have you noticed how Ahab has *humbled himself before me*?' (1 Ki. 21:29).

David declares: '*I . . . humbled myself with fasting*' (Ps. 35:13).

The Old Testament was originally written in Hebrew, so it is important to discover the original meaning of its expressions. In Hebrew, the root of the word 'to fast' – *ana* – is the same as that of the word 'to humble oneself'. Thus fasting is inseparable from humbling oneself.

Jesus gives precise instructions about fasting: 'When you fast, put oil on your head and wash your face, so that it will not be obvious to men that you are fasting, but only to your Father who is unseen' (Mt. 6:17-18).

We can conclude that, in the Bible, fasting is the outward sign of an inward attitude. It denotes an attitude of humility, of dependence and of complete surrender to God. Fasting expresses a desire to break momentarily with our habitual behaviour, for example eating, and to replace it with something even better and even more important: the presence of God, the Word of God.

Fasting is like swimming upstream

Fasting does not come naturally to us – it is like swimming against the current.

A baby puts everything in its mouth: it does not care whether it is good or bad, clean or dirty. Twentieth-century man acts the same way: in order to secure himself against the future, he crams not only his stomach but also his brain, his mind, his life, his house and his bank account with things and ideas that might help and protect him.

The desire to take something and fill oneself with it contributed to bringing sin into the world: 'When the woman saw that the fruit of the tree was good for food . . . she took some and ate it' (Ge. 3:6).

Fasting involves refusing this desire.

Prayer and fasting: a battle

Fasting, accompanied by prayer, is a way of sharpening our weapons for spiritual warfare.

'Prayer is one of the main battlefields where spiritual combat takes place.'[1]

'To deny the reality of the devil's presence in our spiritual lives is to open them up to his activity.'[2]

'The devil knows that prayer is one of the key strategies of the believer, his vital breath. So his constant efforts to make us neglect this activity should not surprise us. In C.S. Lewis' book *The Screwtape Letters*, he describes in a masterly way how obsessed the Evil One is with destroying the Christian's prayer-life.'[3]

The devil never gives up!

Many of us often feel something like a mysterious force impelling us not to pray. Never forget the reality expressed in Ephesians 6:12 – 'Our fight is not against any physical enemy . . . we are up against the unseen power that controls this dark world.'

When we practise fasting and prayer, we proclaim openly to God and to the powers of darkness that we are not relying on our personal resources – our own strength and intelligence – but on the help and intervention of God. We are turning to the Lord in an attitude of dependence and total surrender.

Jehoshaphat expressed this attitude perfectly when 'a vast army' was preparing to attack him (2 Ch. 20:2–12). How did he react? He proclaimed a fast for all Judah and called upon all the people to seek help from the Lord. Listen to his beautiful prayer:

'We have no power to face this vast army that is attacking us. We do not know what to do, but our eyes are upon you' (v. 12).

Jehoshaphat could have appointed a committee, defined objectives, planned a strategy, drawn up an organization chart, strengthened his army, and launched an immediate counter-attack. Instead, he fasted and prayed . . . We learn subsequently that the Lord himself fought for Jehoshaphat and won the victory (2 Ch. 20:22).

We have to face it: fasting is not natural: it goes against the grain. However, it is one way of taking a stand in the spiritual battle.

Never forget that in spiritual warfare prayer is a powerful weapon which can be 'sharpened' by the practice of fasting.

One of the opposition forces we encounter in the spiritual battle is human nature: it just does not like prayer! That is one reason why the disciples went to sleep during a prayer meeting. Jesus told them: 'Your spirit is willing, but human nature is weak' (Mt. 26:41).

In spiritual warfare, our soul and mind both need to be fit and at 'top-level' for us to be available to God.

As I write these lines, the Olympic Games are taking place at Atlanta in the USA. I am following attentively the competitions in the different disciplines. According to the TV commentator, each athlete has trained during the last four years for at least six hours a day. Their meals, their sleep and all their activities outside of sport have been carefully regulated. In addition, if they want to win, they must furnish a sustained effort up to the last minute. In a wrestling match, one athlete dominated his opponent right from the beginning; however, four seconds before the final gong, he allowed himself to be surprised by his opponent who pinned him to the canvas.

Martin Luther used to say that he practised fasting to keep a tight rein on his body.

'One of the purposes and benefits of fasting is to crucify the flesh and liberate the spirit to seek God.'[4]

The apostle Paul wrote about the need to master the body:

'I run the race with determination. I am no shadow-boxer, I really fight! I am my body's sternest master, for fear that when I have preached to others I should myself be disqualified' (1 Co. 9:26–27).

These words could be paraphrased as follows: 'I don't run blindly in all directions, but I keep in the prescribed track and never lose sight of the finishing tape. I don't box against shadows, but I discipline and train my body so that it obeys me perfectly. I want to master it completely lest, after calling others to join in the competition and after telling them the rules, I find myself disqualified!'

True, Paul does not mention fasting in this passage. Nonetheless, since we are soul, mind and body, spiritual warfare requires also our body to be fit.

Someone has said: 'Those who overcome Satan are those who succeed in keeping their bodies and their physical appetites in submission to God.'

For more than twenty-five years, I have gone for a run every morning, come rain or shine . . . or snow. Twice a week I run at the stadium – not because I love running but because I know I must keep my body under control. When I feel fit physically, it is easier for me to pray.

Before starting a lecture on theology, Spurgeon used to require his students to recite the multiplication tables in order to keep their minds alert. Perhaps you prefer maths to jogging? It's up to you!

Other definitions and quotations

Though the word 'fast' has the same root in Hebrew as the word 'humble oneself', it also means 'to decorate with ribbons', in other words it is a way of dressing up the soul before receiving the visit of her Beloved.

Le Sens du Jeûne. Ed. Pneumathèque

Fasting in the Bible generally means going without all food and drink for a period (e.g. Est. 4:16), and not merely refraining from certain foods.

The New Bible Dictionary. IVP

The act of total or partial abstinence from food for a limited period of time, usually undertaken for moral or religious reasons.

Evangelical Dictionary of Theology

Fasting is not so much a question of rejecting one's pleasures as of exchanging one pleasure for another.

Fasting both gives us time to pray and allows other people to eat instead of us. The voluntary privation of the rich becomes the necessary abundance of the poor.

Augustine

Public or private fasting is an outward witness to an inward affliction.

Fasting expresses an inward affliction of the heart. It is a way of expressing to God our real grief concerning ourselves and our sins, with a genuine humility springing from the fear of God.

Calvin

True fasting is not a purely outward activity: it implies renouncing evil and forbidden pleasures (Isaiah 58:1–3).

Nouveau Dictionnaire Biblique, Ed. Emmaüs

Fasting means voluntarily consuming only water during a certain period. This definition implies two factors:

- *a physiological factor: it is a sudden interruption of the usual rhythm of meals which completely deprives the organism of all food, solid or liquid, during a certain time. (Any amount of water may be drunk as it is not food.)*

- *a psychological factor: it is a voluntary act freely undertaken, whatever the motivation of this radical refusal to satisfy a fundamental human need.*

A doctor

21

It is the exercise of a personal, physical and spiritual discipline by means of complete or partial abstinence from food and/or drink for a spiritual purpose. Isaiah 58 shows that the spiritual aspect of fasting is so important that without it the physical aspect is meaningless.

Dr Homer Payne

Fasting is the interruption of the normal rhythm of meals. On the one hand, it breaks the usual rhythm of eating, and on the other, it reduces the amount of food consumed during a certain time.

J. Trémolières

Fasting is a way of showing God our real priorities: thereby we tell God that eternal values are more important to us than temporal ones, and that spiritual values have priority over physical and material needs.

Ian Newberry

Fasting is a way of humbling ourselves before God in order to open ourselves deeply to the Word of God and await with confidence his intervention in our life.

Ian Newberry

ANSWERS
TO THE TEST
ON PAGE 18

	RIGHT	WRONG	DON'T KNOW
1. In the Bible, fasting is mentioned 8 times; it is practised by 5 people in exceptional circumstances.		X	
2. In the Bible, the word 'fasting' can mean 'humbling oneself before God'.	X		
3. Jesus practised fasting, but he did not explain how or why one should fast.		X	
4. Isaiah 58 deals with right and wrong motives for fasting.	X		
5. Group fasting was often practised in the Old Testament, but never in the New Testament.		X	
6. In the Bible, fasting was always practised with a view to obtaining an answer to prayer.		X	
7. In Scripture, God himself speaks about fasting.	X		
8. The Bible refers to fasting more than seventy times.	X		

5. Questions for further reflection

a. Why did you buy this book about the biblical teaching on fasting?

_____

_____

b. What questions about the practice of fasting do you have at present?

_____

_____

c. Have you already practised fasting? If so, for what reason? If not, do you know personally someone who practises fasting? Why does he or she practise fasting?

_____

_____

_____

_____

_____

_____

d. Do you agree with the author that 'prayer is a battle'?

_____

- What is the nature of this battle? See Ephesians 6:11–12

_____

_____

- What do you do when you don't want to pray, or when you find it hard to pray?

_____

_____

- Do you agree that spiritual warfare requires that body, mind and soul be kept fit? If so, what are you doing specifically in order to keep fit in each of these areas?

_____

_____

_____

e. Re-read 1 Kings 21:29 and 2 Chronicles 20:2–12, then write down your personal definition of fasting as it was practised in the Bible.

_____

_____

_____

f. Read Isaiah 58:1–14, try to complete the table below by listing the differences between the right way to fast and the wrong way.

The right way to fast	The wrong way to fast

g. The same text, Isaiah 58:1–14, mentions the blessings that accompany fasting. List the spiritual benefits of practising fasting in the right way.

_____

_____

_____

_____

_____

_____

Reflection

_____

_____

_____

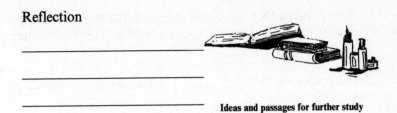

Ideas and passages for further study

_____

Prayer

_____

_____

_____

_____

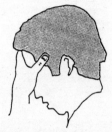

Ideas for strengthening and deepening my prayer-life

_____

Action

_____

_____

_____

_____

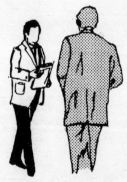

Ideas to put into practice

_____

CHAPTER 2 FASTING IN THE BIBLE

1. A panoramic view of fasting in the Bible

2. Biblical passages which mention fasting

3. Four basic truths concerning fasting in the Bible

   A. Fasting must always be accompanied by prayer
   B. Fasting is a gesture of self-humbling
   C. Fasting is a gesture of solidarity
   D. Fasting must always be accompanied by the Word of God

4. The differences between the right and wrong ways to fast

   A. The wrong way to fast
   - Fasting superficially
   - Fasting ostentatiously
   - Fasting to mortify the flesh
   - The wrong approach to fasting: a warning

   B. The right way to fast
   - The teaching of Jesus
   - The teaching of Isaiah

5. Questions for further reflection

Fasting in the right way is an excellent practice: it gladdens the heart and pleases God.

Hermas, 'The Shepherd'

1. A panoramic view of fasting in the Bible

– The Old and New Testaments give several examples of individual and group fasting.

– The prophets warn about fasting in the wrong way.

– Jesus explains clearly why and how we should fast.

– Paul warns against fanaticism in the area of fasting.

– The early church shows how we should fast today.

2. Biblical passages which mention fasting

I was surprised to discover more than seventy references to fasting in the Bible. I encourage you not only to read these passages, but to consider them in their historical context. Some of these fasts were approved by God, of others God disapproved.

Here are the passages in the Old Testament that mention fasting:

Ge. 24:33   Abraham's servant goes to look for a wife for Isaac, Abraham's, son. He fasts until his mission is accomplished.

Ex. 34:28	When Moses receives the tables of the Law written by God himself, he abstains from eating and drinking during a period of forty days and forty nights.
Lev. 16:19–31	God tells Moses that all the people should humble themselves by fasting on the Day of Atonement.
Lev. 23:14	God forbids eating roasted or new grain during this annual fast.
Lev. 23:26–32	God appoints a sacred assembly to be celebrated on this day of fasting.
Nu. 6:3–4	The partial fast of the Nazirite.
Nu. 29:7	How to fast on the Day of Atonement: by humbling oneself.
Dt. 9:9	Moses abstains for forty days from eating and drinking on Mt. Sinai when God gives the tables of the Law.
Dt. 9:18	Moses again fasts for forty days when he returns to Mt. Sinai after breaking the tables of the Law because of the idolatry of the people of Israel.
Jdg. 20:26	At Bethel, Israel fasts before the Lord in order to know his will: 'Shall we go up again to battle with Benjamin?' They also fast out of gratitude.
1 Sam. 1:7–8	Desperate to have a child, Hannah fasts to express her grief.

1 Sam. 7:5–6	Samuel and all Israel meet at Mizpah to pray, fast and confess their sins.
1 Sam. 14:24–30	Saul orders his soldiers to fast until he has avenged himself of his enemies.
1 Sam. 20:34	Jonathan fasts because his father wants to kill his best friend, David.
1 Sam. 28:20–23	After consulting a witch at Endor, Saul fasts all day and all night.
1 Sam. 30:11–12	An Egyptian goes without food for three days: an involuntary fast in wartime.
1 Sam. 31:13	After the defeat of Israel by the Philistines and the suicide of Saul, the men of Jabesh Gilead bury his body and fast for seven days.
2 Sam. 3:35	David fasts after the death of Abner.
2 Sam. 11:11	Uriah refuses to eat while Israel is at war.
2 Sam. 1:12	David and his men fast all day after learning of Saul's death.
2 Sam. 12:16	David fasts when his son falls ill.
1 Ki. 13:8–24	God orders a man of God to fast. He disobeys . . . and is eaten by a lion.

1 Ki. 19:8	Elijah fasts during his forty-day journey to Horeb.
1 Ki. 21:4–5	When Naboth refuses Ahab's demand, in anger the king starts a fast.
1 Ki. 21:9	Jezebel proclaims a day of fasting in order to mask her sin.
1 Ki. 21:27	After Nathan points out his sin, Ahab fasts and humbles himself before God.
1 Ch. 10:12	Saul's valiant men fast for seven days.
2 Ch. 20:3–13	When the enemy prepares to attack Judah, Jehoshaphat proclaims a fast for all the people.
Ezr. 8:21–23	Ezra and all the people pray and fast in order to implore God to protect them.
Ezr. 10:6	Ezra fasts because of the unfaithfulness of the exiles.
Ne. 1:4	Nehemiah mourns, fasts and prays when he learns that Jerusalem is broken down and that the people are in great trouble and disgrace.
Ne. 9:1–3	The people fast to confess their sins following the reading of the Law and worship.
Est. 4:3	Mordecai and the Jews fast when they learn of Haman's plan to destroy them.

Est. 4:16	Esther fasts three days and nights.
Est. 9:20–31	Mordecai and Esther appoint the feast of Purim to celebrate the intervention of God in favour of the Jewish people. Their sorrow is turned into joy and their mourning into celebration.
Job 33:19–20	Job fasts involuntarily while ill since he finds food repulsive.
Ps. 35:13	David fasts when his friends are ill.
Ps. 42:3	Their tears are the sole food of the sons of Korah.
Ps. 69:10	David fasts when he seeks deliverance from his enemies.
Ps. 102:4	The psalmist is so miserable that he forgets to eat.
Ps. 107:18	The foolish are so rebellious that their guilt feelings cause them to lose their appetite for food.
Ps 109:24	David's knees are weakened by fasting.
Isa. 58:1–13	Right and wrong ways to fast are contrasted.
Jer. 14:12	God refuses to hear the prayers of his people because of their wickedness: 'Although they fast, I will not listen to their cry . . .'

Jer. 36:6	Jeremiah tells Baruch that on the day of fasting he must read the words of the Lord to the people in the temple.
Jer. 36:9	Jehoiakim proclaims a fast at Jerusalem for all the people of Judah.
Da. 1:12–16	Daniel and his friends refuse to defile themselves with royal food and wine.
Da. 6:18	King Darius fasts while Daniel is in the den of lions.
Da. 9:3	Daniel fasts in order to devote himself wholly to prayer. This fast is accompanied by a wonderful prayer (9–14).
Da. 10:3	Daniel mourns and fasts for three weeks, abstaining from meat and wine.
Joel 1:14–20	In time of drought and famine, Joel calls upon the people to fast.
Joel 2:12	The Lord calls upon the people to return wholeheartedly to him with fasting, weeping and mourning.
Joel 2:15	A national fast is called by the sound of a trumpet.
Jnh. 3:5–10	The king and the people of Nineveh believe God and declare a fast as an expression of repentance.

Zec. 7:5   God asks his people: 'When you fasted and mourned in the fifth and seventh months for the past seventy years, was it really for me that you fasted?'

Zec. 8:19   When the Exile was over, four fast-days were turned into joyful festivals.

To summarize:

We now seek to understand the overall and underlying significance of fasting in the Old Testament.

The occasions and reasons for fasting are varied. In general, fasting that is approved by God is an expression of humility before God. The soul needs to express itself by means of physical attitudes and actions.

In fasting, people turn to the Lord (Da. 9:3; Ezr. 8:21) in an attitude of dependence and total surrender: before undertaking a difficult task (Jdg. 20:26; Est. 4:16; Ne. 1:4); in order to plead for healing (2 Sam. 12:16–22) or for forgiveness after committing a fault (1 Ki. 21:27); in order to mourn someone's death (1 Sam. 31:13; 2 Sam. 1:12), to lament a national misfortune (1 Sam. 7:6; 2 Sam. 1:12) or to bring a natural disaster to an end (Joel 2:12–17).

In the Old Testament, fasting accompanied by prayer expresses an attitude of faith and dependence in which one opens oneself to the Word of God and awaits his intervention. It is a declaration of dependence on God. All of this is summed up in the beautiful prayer of Jehoshaphat while fasting:

'We have no power to face this vast army . . . but our eyes are upon you' (2 Ch. 20:12).

Fasting in the New Testament

Mt. 4:2   Led by the Spirit into the desert to be
                 tempted, Jesus fasts during forty days
                 and forty nights.

Mt. 6:16–18   Jesus teaches about how to practise
                 fasting.

Mt. 9:14–15   The disciples of John the Baptist ask
                 Jesus why his disciples do not fast.

Mt. 9:15   Jesus says that the time to fast will be
                 when the bridegroom is taken away.

Mt. 11:18   John the Baptist practises fasting.

Mt. 15:32   Jesus refuses to send the crowd home
                 with nothing to eat.

Mt. 17:21*   Jesus teaches that prayer and fasting are
                 necessary in order to expel certain
                 demons.

Mk. 2:18–19   Why the disciples of Jesus do not
                 practise fasting.

Mk. 9:29*   'Nothing can drive out this kind of [evil
                 spirit] except prayer and fasting.'

Lk. 2:37   Anna, the prophetess, worships God
                 day and night with fasting and prayers.

Lk 4:2   Led by the Spirit to spend forty days in
                 the desert, Jesus practises fasting.

Lk. 5:33–35	Why don't the disciples of Jesus fast?
Lk. 7:33	John the Baptist practises fasting.
Lk. 18:12	The Pharisee prays: 'I fast twice a week . . .'
Ac. 9:9	After his conversion, Paul neither eats nor drinks for three days.
Ac. 10:30*	Cornelius prays and fasts, then an angel speaks to him.
Ac. 13:2–3	The church at Antioch prays and fasts before sending out Barnabas and Paul.
Ac. 14.23	At Lystra, the church prays and fasts when appointing elders.
Ac. 23:12–21	Some Jews decide to eat nothing until they succeed in killing Paul.
Ac. 27:9	An allusion to Jewish fasting on the Day of Atonement.
Ac. 27:33	Paul tells the crew: 'For a fortnight now you've had no food.'
1 Co. 7:5*	Another form of fasting is abstinence from marital relations in order to devote oneself wholly to prayer.
1 Co. 8:13	Paul recommends abstinence from eating or drinking, if necessary, to avoid causing a brother to stumble.

2 Co. 6:5	Paul tells of having to endure being flogged and imprisoned, and having to work like a slave and to go without food.
2 Co. 11:27	Paul says he has known hunger and doing without meals on many occasions.
1 Ti. 4:3	False prophets will impose abstinence from certain kinds of food.

* In these verses, certains manuscripts mention fasting as well as prayer, but scholars specializing in the study of the many copies available of the New Testament books generally agree that fasting was added to the original text at a later period when asceticism came into vogue in the early church.

A. Kuen

What does God think about fasting?

After reading all these passages in the Old and New Testaments, it is interesting that it is often God who takes the initiative in the matter of fasting. For example, the annual fast mentioned in Leviticus 23:20–31 was instigated by God. On other occasions, God invites his people to return to him with all their heart, by fasting (Joel 2:12).

Moved by God, prophets, and sometimes kings, proclaim a national fast, a practical way of bringing the people together in order to turn their attention away from idols.

God sees the person who fasts and he knows their real motivations. 'Have you noticed how Ahab has humbled himself before me?' (1 Ki. 21:27). 'Although they fast, I will not listen to their cry . . .' (Jer.14:12). 'When you fasted . . . , was it really for me that you fasted?' (Zec. 7:5).

In his gospel, Luke, a doctor, mentions specifically that Jesus was led *by the Spirit* into the desert where he fasted for forty days (Lk. 4:1–2).

In the book of Acts, it was while the church at Antioch was fasting and praying that God spoke by his Holy Spirit and gave the instruction: 'Set Barnabas and Saul apart for me for a task to which I have called them' (Ac. 13:2).

So we can affirm that God – the Father, the Son and the Holy Spirit – sometimes called on people to practise fasting.

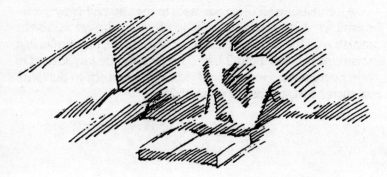

3. Four basic truths concerning fasting in the Bible

A. Fasting must always be accompanied by prayer

In the Bible, both individual and collective fasting are always accompanied by prayer.

Individual fasting
- Moses (Ex. 34:28)
- Elijah (1 Ki. 19:8)
- Nehemiah (Ne. 1:4)
- Jesus (Mt. 6:1–18)
- Anna (Lk. 2:37)

Collective fasting
- Samuel and the people of Israel (1 Sam 7:5-6)
- Jehoshaphat and the people of Judah (2 Ch. 20:3)
- Esther and the Jews (Est. 4:16)
- The church at Antioch (Ac. 13:1–4)

The practical lesson for us:

We advise you always to accompany fasting with prayer. In the book of Nehemiah, we see how the fasting people of God were fed by passages from the Bible and by prayer (Ne. 8 and 9). Read passages from God's Word during your fast, and use them as a basis and as an inspiration for your prayers.

B. Fasting is a gesture of self-humbling

In the Word of God, fasting often expresses inward sorrow and humility before God.

When looking up references to fasting in the Old Testament, we need to take into account synonymous expressions like 'deny yourselves' (NIV – other versions: 'humble yourselves') in Leviticus 16:29, Numbers 29:7, etc.

- Ahab humbles himself before God and confesses his sin (1 Ki. 21:29).

- Esdras and the people fast and confess their sins to God (1 Esd. 9:1).

- David prays and weeps because of the death of his child (2 Sam. 12:22).

The practical lesson for us:

My actions or my words may have grieved the Spirit of God. By fasting and confession, I can express to God my sorrow and my desire for forgiveness.

By fasting, I express to God with my body the sorrow I feel about my sin. This 'godly sorrow' is positive: it produces first repentance, then happiness and joy. This is what the Lord Almighty says: 'The fasts of the fourth, fifth, seventh and tenth months will become joyful and glad occasions and happy festivals for Judah' (Zec. 8:19). To humble ourselves under the mighty hand of God is a necessary and positive process which brings blessing both to ourselves and to those around us.

Realizing the gravity of sin, then firmly resisting the sin that dogs our feet is absolutely essential. Fasting helps us to express and strengthen our determination – with God's help – to walk the path of sanctification.

However, we need to be perfectly clear: fasting in itself does not purify us from sin: only the blood of Christ can do that.

C. Fasting is a gesture of solidarity

Fasting can also accompany an attitude of solidarity which expresses itself by hospitality, generosity and practical compassion.

Isa. 58:7   (After speaking about true and false fasting) 'Share your food with the hungry . . . provide the poor wanderer with shelter . . . when you see the naked . . . clothe him, and [do] not turn away from your own flesh and blood?'

Mt. 6:1–18   Jesus mentions three things to be practised in secret: giving, praying and fasting.

'The first Christians were not content to give their surplus. When someone was going hungry, they fasted for two or three days in order to give him what they had intended to eat themselves. In other words, they gave what they had to live on.'[5]

The practical lesson for us:

Fasting out of solidarity reminds us that intimacy with God on the one hand, and communication, communion and sharing with our neighbour on the other, are inseparable. Augustine, who often practised this kind of fasting, stated: 'In fasting out of solidarity, the voluntary privation of the rich becomes the necessary abundance of the poor . . . Fasting both permits others to eat instead of us and also gives us more time to pray.'

A Christian organization put out a beautiful poster representing a European family at table with an extra place laid and the following words: 'Add an extra place to your table!' Let us be prompt to share with those – in Africa or in India, in Romania or the Philippines etc. – who are prevented from eating normally. Why not go without a meal in order to give the money saved for those in need?

'When we fast, we should not keep the uneaten food for ourselves, but instead give it away to others.'[6]

D. Fasting must always be accompanied by the Word of God

'The Word of God must reform and refashion not only our lives but also our prayers.'[7]

Augustine said: 'Fasting raises the spirit toward heavenly food.'

In the Bible, fasting, prayer and the Word of God are closely linked. In Nehemiah 9:1–3, the people of God meet to 'celebrate a fast' – note the expression! They confess their sins and listen to the reading of the book of the Law. A quarter of the day is devoted to the reading of the Word of God. There is the spring and the root of all true revival. In chapters 8 and 9, note how thirsty the people are for God's Word. Even children – old enough to understand – are present and paying attention (Ne. 8:3). What a magnificent scene: all the people assembled are in the city square to listen to the public reading of Holy Scripture!

I would like to point out briefly three other Bible characters who read or listened to the Word of God during their fast:

Daniel	While Daniel is fasting and praying, he receives the visit of the angel Gabriel (Da. 9:21) who declares the Word of God to him and urges him to pay attention to it (9:3–23).
Jeremiah	Jeremiah gives Baruch the following instructions: 'Go to the house of the Lord on a day of fasting. Read to the people from the scroll the words of the Lord that you wrote as I dictated.' (Jer. 36:6).
Jesus	Jesus, himself the Word of God (John 1:1), practises and teaches fasting. He quotes the Word of God, using it to refute the devil who is seeking to cast doubt on his deity. 'It is written . . . it is written . . . it is written . . .' The Word is his food, his strength, his sword to fight and rout the enemy! (Lk. 4:1–13).

These passages and examples illustrate how important it is to 'nourish' our time of fasting by meditating, reading and studying God's Word. His Word will prevent us from falling into sheer mysticism, put the devil to flight and sweep away unbelief (Lk. 4:13). It will keep us in the centre of God's will (Job 23:12) and make our prayers powerful and effective (Jn 15:7–8).

Listen to the testimony of George Muller who read right through the Bible more than 150 times:

'For more than fourteen years, I have devoted myself daily to the reading of the Word of God. I read, meditate and study the Word. Through this reading my heart is comforted, encouraged, warmed, instructed and sometimes corrected and warned. Through my reading, I obtain food for my soul. The

Word then sets my heart ablaze in a prayer of confession, thanksgiving and intercession.'

In his book *How to Pray*, the Scottish pastor and theologian Graham Scroggie (1877–1958) has this to say about the importance of the Word of God and prayer:

'For too long, prayer and Bible study have been divorced, and with sad results. What God has joined together, we should never separate.

'Do not spend time in prayer first, before spending time in the Word. The order is important: first the Word, then prayer. For the Word is the means by which prayer is conceived and the vehicle by which it is expressed – and not the other way round.'

Feeding on the Word of God while fasting, enables us to experience the reality stated by Jesus: 'Man shall not live by bread alone, but by every word that proceeds out of the mouth of God' (Mt. 4:4).

'Food does not sustain us; God sustains us. In Christ "all things hold together" (Col 1:17). Therefore, in experiences of fasting, we are not so much abstaining from food as we are feasting on the Word of God.'[8]

Listen to this beautiful prayer:

'Your Word is like water. Refresh us at its spring, dip us in its stream, carry us down to its sea. Your Word is like a fire. May it illumine us, without dazzling us. May it warm us, without burning us. May it set us ablaze, without consuming us. Your Word is like the heavens. May it enlarge our minds so that we may know something of the height and depth of all things. Your Word is like the earth. May we become so deeply rooted in it that we feel the solidity and the durability of all that you give, demand and promise. Amen.'[9]

Let's now summarize these four great truths. We should fast with prayer, fast to express our humility before God, fast and share with those in need, and above all fast and feed our soul on the strong meat of the Word of God. If we base our prayers on the Scriptures, they will become reality!

4. The differences between the right and wrong ways to fast

The Bible mentions two different kinds of fasting. The following table will enable you to see at a glance the differences between the kind of fasting which pleases God and the kind which is quite useless.

Wrong ways to fast	Right ways to fast
Fasting because we are angry with God. Isa. 58:4	Fasting to please God, not ourselves. Zec. 7:5
Fasting for one's personal glory. Jer. 14:12–14	Fasting in order to feed on God's Word and presence. Mt. 4:4
Fasting to be seen by others. Mt. 6:18	Fasting in secret to be seen only by God. Mt. 6:18
Fasting out of a legalistic tradition (Israel had fasted during the previous seventy years.) Zec. 7:1–5	Fasting to obtain strength. After fasting, Jesus was clothed with the power of the Spirit. Lk. 4:14
Fasting without understanding its biblical meaning. Zec. 7:5	Fasting, before all else, in order to meet with God. Personal desires and exceptional circumstances are secondary. Mt. 6:16–17; Isa. 58

Wrong ways to fast	Right ways to fast
Fasting out of asceticism – denying the desires of the body in order to gain merit. 1 Ti. 4:3	Fasting in an attitude of dependence and availability before God. 1 Ch . 20:1–12
Fasting in the attempt to put pressure on God in order to force him to do what I want. Fasting then becomes a sort of hunger strike. Isa. 58:4	Fasting and praying in order to submit my will to God's will and to accept his plans for my life. Jer. 29:11

'For I know the plans I have for you,' declares the Lord, 'plans to prosper you and not to harm you, plans to give you a hope and a future. Then you will call upon me and come and pray to me, and I will listen to you.

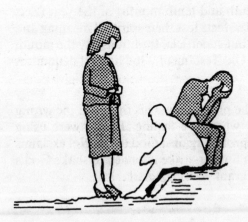

You will seek me and find me when you seek me with all your heart.' (Jer. 29:11–13)

49

A. The wrong way to fast

'Fasting is a useless and even dangerous remedy for those who do not understand why and how to practise it.'

John Chrysostom

Warnings about unbiblical ways of fasting

The wrong kind of fasting means fasting for purposes which are not taught in the Scriptures.

The annual fast prescribed by the Law of Moses took place once a year (Lev. 16:29–32). All who belonged to the people of God were obliged to observe this fast. On that day, they had to abstain from their daily work and take part in the sacred assembly. It was a day of atonement, of confession, of repentance, and a day for the people to humble themselves before God (Nu. 29.7–11).

After the Exile, four other fasts were prescribed: those of the fourth, fifth, seventh and tenth months of the year (Zec. 7:5; 8:19). In time, these fasts lost their spiritual meaning and became merely pious but superficial traditions. By the mouth of his prophets in the Old Testament, God himself denounces this superficiality.

In Isaiah 58:1–5, the prophet puts his finger on the wrong motivations of those who were fasting. People were using fasting as a means of protest against God (v. 4). No! exclaims Isaiah, fasting is not a hunger-strike intended to shake God's determination not to grant your requests!

God is not an unmoveable block of marble who can only be brought to change his mind by so many days of fasting. Biblical fasting is not a kind of 'token' we put in a slot in order to obtain something from God. Rather, as we humble ourselves before God and acknowledge our weakness, he gives us strength to change our attitudes to others by loving them in practical ways such as forgiving them, welcoming them into our home and sharing with them.

In Isaiah's view, the people of God had:

the right outward motions . . but the wrong inward attitudes
the right theory . . . . but the wrong practice
the right appearance . . . . . but the wrong motivation.

God did not wish even to listen to these people who refused to quit their evil ways – and still less to answer their prayers!

The practical lesson for us:

It is important for us to analyse the reasons why we fast. Fasting must always be accompanied by humbling ourselves in prayer, taking our rightful place before our great, holy and sovereign God.

Biblical fasting is not a feat of asceticism. Its purpose is not to get us into an exalted psychological or religious mood. As you will learn at the end of this manual, throughout the history of the church, certain people who devoted much time to fasting nevertheless drifted slowly away from the truths of the Bible.

Before beginning our fast, we could pray in the following words:

'Search me, O God, and know my heart; test me and know my anxious thoughts. See if there is any offensive way in me and lead me in the way everlasting.' (Ps. 139:23–24)

Fasting superficially

Superficiality is one of the curses of the present day. Superficial people do not delve deeply into things. They are quite satisfied with appearances – with the wrappings. Jesus attacked and denounced the superficiality of the Pharisees:

'Blind Pharisee! First clean the inside of the cup and dish, and then the outside also will be clean' (Mt. 23:26).

By the mouth of Jeremiah, God declares that he turns a deaf ear to the prayers of such people:

'Although they fast, I will not listen to their cry' (Jer. 14:12).

Why is God not pleased by this kind of fasting? Because of . . .

- their great backsliding (v. 7),
- the lies of the false prophets (v. 14).

The prophet Zechariah asks the fundamental question concerning the real motivations of the people who were fasting in a legalistic way:

'When you fasted and mourned in the fifth and seventh months for the past seventy years, was it really for me that you fasted?' (Zec. 7:5).

For seventy years the people had kept up a tradition to which they were slaves. Though this practice had originally been valuable, it had degenerated into a dry, hard legalism, void of the presence and power of God.

We should fast not to please ourselves or others, but to please God.

The practical lesson for us:

We need to be honest and transparent before God. It is better not to fast than to do so simply to please others, and without a deep and sincere conviction based on the Word of God.

Other examples of unbiblical fasting

Saul practised fasting in the wrong way (1 Sam 14:24). Not only did he try to force the people to fast with him, but his fast was begun out of anger and jealousy, and with the determination to avenge himself against his enemies.

Jezebel asked the elders of Naboth's home-town to proclaim a collective fast and to invite Naboth to take part in it so that he could be falsely accused of having cursed God and the king and then be put to death (1 Ki. 21:9).

Why do you think the Pharisees fasted on Mondays and Thursdays? Because they were market days – and so there would be crowds of 'spectators' to admire them!

Luke 18:11–12 mentions specifically that the Pharisee in the parable prayed 'with [or to] himself'. As a result the Pharisee's fasting was quite useless. All that interested him was going through the motions and keeping up outward appearances – whereas God looks at the heart (1 Sam. 16:7).

Fasting ostentatiously

Jesus teaches that fasting loses its meaning when it is practised in full view of others in order to win their admiration: 'Just see how spiritual I am!'

'When you fast, brush your hair and wash your face so that nobody knows you are fasting!' (Mt. 6:17–18).

Fasting to mortify the flesh

The apostle Paul rejected asceticism with its disdain for the body.

'Why . . . do you take the slightest notice of those purely human prohibitions – "Don't touch this," "Don't taste that" and "Don't handle the other"? "This" "that" and "the other" will all pass away after use! I know that these regulations look wise with their self-inspired efforts at worship, their policy of self-humbling, and their studied neglect of the body. But in actual practice they do honour, not to God, but to man's own pride' (Col. 2:21–23).

UNBIBLICAL FASTING

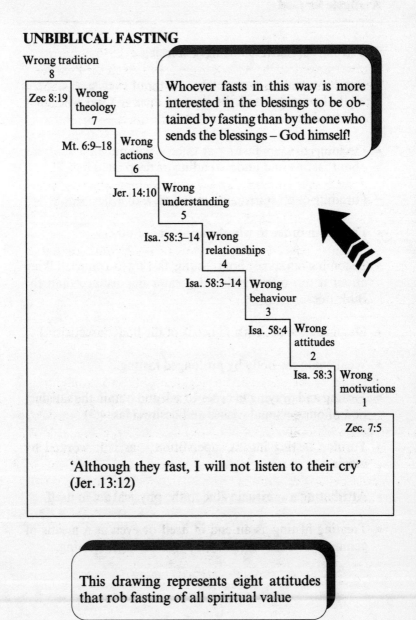

Wrong tradition
8

Zec 8:19 | Wrong theology
7

Mt. 6:9–18 | Wrong actions
6

Whoever fasts in this way is more interested in the blessings to be obtained by fasting than by the one who sends the blessings – God himself!

Jer. 14:10 | Wrong understanding
5

Isa. 58:3–14 | Wrong relationships
4

Isa. 58:3–14 | Wrong behaviour
3

Isa. 58:4 | Wrong attitudes
2

Isa. 58:3 | Wrong motivations
1

Zec. 7:5

'Although they fast, I will not listen to their cry' (Jer. 13:12)

This drawing represents eight attitudes that rob fasting of all spiritual value

55

The wrong approach to fasting: a warning

- Rejecting fasting completely – without ever studying the biblical passages and the lives of men of God who have practised fasting.

- Deciding to start fasting at once – without first studying about fasting and understanding its deep meaning.

- Parading one's spirituality in full view of other people.

- Fasting in order to win the approval of others.

- Becoming fanatical about fasting: fasting too much, talking about it too often, giving it greater importance than the Bible does.

- Despising the desires and needs of the body (asceticism).

- Weakening the body by prolonged fasting.

- Fasting and praying in order to ask and obtain the satisfaction of our personal wishes and desires (Jas. 4:3).

- Turning fasting into a superstition – as if it worked by magic.

- Attributing a spiritual value to the physical act in itself.

- Treating fasting as an end in itself or even as a means of gaining merit and automatically obtaining a blessing.

- Believing that fasting is a means of salvation.

- Believing that prayer and fasting compel God to give one spiritual power.

- Considering fasting as automatically conferring the ability to receive revelations from God, to expiate one's sins, to purify oneself spiritually, to protect oneself against evil spirits etc.

- Trying to 'empty' oneself by fasting in order to 'be filled' with a mystical experience of an ecstatic character.

- Treating fasting as a legal obligation – forcing oneself and other people to practise fasting.

- Fasting rigidly at set times – and then becoming fearful about not respecting them.

Some important remarks:

Both personal and collective fasting must be voluntary acts. Never force other people to practise fasting. In a way, fasting is like sleeping: the harder you try, the less you succeed! It is so important to approach fasting in the right way: we need to be able to fast joyfully – because we understand why we are fasting and because we really want to fast.

Fasting is in no way a means of getting our sins forgiven; only the blood of Christ can purify us of every sin (1 Jn. 1:7). Nor is it by fasting that God indwells us by his Holy Spirit (Ac. 2:38). Fasting is above all a way of expressing in a definite way our hunger and thirst for God, for his presence and for his Word (Ps. 42:1–3).

B. The right way to fast

The teaching of Jesus

Matthew 4:1–2: 'Then Jesus was led by the Spirit up into the desert, to be tempted by the devil. After a fast of forty days and forty nights he was very hungry.'

Before beginning his public ministry, Jesus fasts and prays (Mt. 4:2). In other words, his contact with his Father is his foremost priority. It comes before all else – teaching, training his disciples, performing miracles. Jesus expresses this well in John 4:34: 'My food is doing the will of him who sent me.' The real food that sustains him is his intimate relationship with God. It is indispensable.

Jesus practises fasting before inaugurating his public ministry with a proclamation of the whole will of God in the Sermon on the Mount.

Matthew 4:1 is the only verse in the gospels which mentions that Jesus practised fasting – but, of course, this does not mean that he did not fast on other occasions.

It is interesting to note that on this occasion Jesus fasted for forty days, as did Moses (Ex. 24:18) and Elijah (1 Ki. 19:8). During this long period of time, only God spoke with them and sustained them. To the devil who came to tempt him, Jesus retorted: 'Man shall not live by bread alone, but by every word that proceeds out of the mouth of God' (Mt. 4:4).

By practising fasting, Jesus teaches us that eternal values are more important than temporal ones, and that spiritual values have priority over material ones.

Jesus teaches about fasting, but on no occasion does he command it or make it obligatory.

In Matthew 6:1–18, Jesus is not replying to the question 'Do we have to fast?' but giving instructions about the right way to fast.

In this chapter, Jesus underlines three aspects of our devotion to God:

Giving (vv. 1–4): our attitude towards others;

Praying (vv. 6–15): our attitude to God;

Fasting (vv. 16–18): our personal discipline.

Jesus treats together these three aspects of Jewish piety: giving, praying and fasting. These three acts hang together logically and are inseparable in the teaching of the Bible:

– *Giving* expresses our solidarity in regard to the poverty of the world around us.

– *Praying* expresses our dependence on God.

– *Fasting* expresses our desire to show God that spiritual values have priority over material ones in our lives, and our determination to keep the body under control and to combat fleshly influences and attitudes (Gal. 5:17).

Immediately after dealing with these three disciplines, Jesus underlines the importance of not being obsessed with material wealth – 'Don't pile up treasures on earth . . . but keep your treasure in heaven' (Mt 6:19–20).

Fasting should involve our whole being and enable our body, mind and soul to engage in prayer.

In the following verses (Mt. 6:19–34), Jesus deals with the intimate heart of personal spirituality: absolute confidence in God, complete dependence on our heavenly Father, giving top priority to seeking the kingdom of God and setting aside earthly worries.

Jesus seems to pass quite abruptly from the spiritual life to practical realities, from treasures in heaven to troubles on earth. The link suggested by this alternation between the spiritual and the material is very important. We have to learn to 'live with our heart in heaven' – all the while 'keeping our feet on the ground'. If we do not maintain this balance, we will either become mystics, detached from the everyday world, or else activists, void of all genuine spiritual strength – the only source of which is a constantly renewed intimacy with God.

By his teaching, Jesus invites us to cultivate a spirituality that is realistic, balanced and practical.

Fasting in order to come closer to God

When Jesus speaks about fasting, his aim is not to abolish it because of its abuses, but to rehabilitate it by giving instructions about the right way to practise it.

Fasting must be God-centred – focussed on God.

In Matthew 6:18, Jesus tells us that we are not to fast in order to be seen by others, but in order to open ourselves up to the presence of God.

'Everything lies naked and exposed before the eyes of him with whom we have to do' (Heb. 4:13).

Fasting practised for selfish reasons or in a hypocritical way has no value whatsoever in the eyes of God.

'Jesus denounces hypocrisy. A hypocrite is one who wears a mask and who, in order to win the approval of other people, acts ostensibly as if he were humbling himself – and he gets his reward' (v. 16). If the outward motions of spirituality do not spring from the heart, they are completely useless! In speaking about hypocrites, Jesus is certainly alluding to the Pharisees. In Luke 18:9–14, he presents the Pharisees as fasting twice a week, yet their heart is bursting with pride! The Lord insists on the need to be discreet. When fasting, one should wash and dress with one's usual care in order to avoid drawing the attention of others to what one is doing and falling into the trap of 'showing off'.[10]

Before God, there is no room for a veneer or for make-up! We must drop the mask. In fasting and praying in the presence of God, I discover how deceitful my heart is. Faced with the holiness of God, jealousy, bitterness and selfishness are uprooted from my heart.

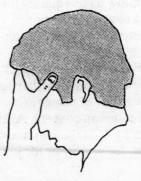

To come before God and to expose ourselves to his presence and his Word expresses our desire to know God and be known by him. In his excellent book *Knowing God*, J. I. Packer explains in a simple but precise way the need and the meaning of such a relationship with God:

'First, knowing God is a matter of *personal dealing*, as is all direct acquaintance with personal beings. Knowing God is more than knowing about Him; it is a matter of dealing with Him as He opens up to you, and being dealt with by Him as He takes knowledge of you . . .

'Second, knowing God is a matter of *personal involvement*, in mind, will, and feeling. It would not, indeed, be a fully personal relationship otherwise. To get to know another person, you have to commit yourself to his company and interests, and be ready to identify yourself with his concerns. Without this, your relationship with him can only be superficial and flavourless.

' "O taste and see that the Lord is good," says the psalmist (Ps. 34:8). To "taste" is, as we say, to "try" a mouthful of something, with a view to appreciating its flavour. A dish may look good, and be well recommended by the cook, but we do not know its real quality till we have tasted it. Similarly, we do not know another person's real quality till we have "tasted" the experience of friendship with him.

'Friends are, so to speak, communicating flavours to each other all the time, by sharing their attitudes both towards each other (think of people in love) and towards everything else that is of common concern. As they thus open their hearts to each other by what they say and do, each "tastes" the quality of the other, for sorrow or for joy . . .

'Then, third, knowing God is a matter of grace. It is a relationship in which the initiative throughout is with God – as it must be, since God is so completely above us and we have so completely forfeited all claim on His favour by our sins. We do not make friends with God; God makes friends with us, bringing us to know Him by making His love known to us . . .

' "Know", when used of God in this way, is a sovereign-grace word, pointing to God's initiative in loving, choosing, redeeming, calling and preserving. That God is fully aware of us "knowing us through and through," as we say, is certainly part of what is meant . . . But it is not the main meaning. The main meaning comes out in passages like the following:

' "And the Lord said to Moses: '. . . I am pleased with you and I know you by your name' " (Ex. 33:17).

' "Before I formed you (Jeremiah) in the womb, I knew you, before you were born I set you apart" (Jer. 1:5).

' "I am the good shepherd; I know my sheep and my sheep know me . . . and I lay down my life for the sheep . . . My sheep listen to my voice; I know them . . . and they shall never perish" (Jn. 10:14f., 27f.).

'Here God's knowledge of those who are His is associated with His whole purpose of saving mercy. It is a knowledge that implies personal affection, redeeming action, covenant faithfulness and providential watchfulness, towards those whom God knows. It implies, in other words, salvation, now and for ever.'

What a joy it is to be in contact with God by prayer: we can tell him everything that is on our hearts and he hears, he listens and he understands.

My deepest motivation to pray lies in God himself. I want to allow myself to be awed by God's presence and to be immersed in his character and attributes. The God whom I encounter so intimately is faithful; eternal, powerful, holy, righteous, personal, all-knowing . . . We need to take care not to imagine that God is like us and to bring him down to our own level. A false image of God makes our prayer-life more difficult.

In order to cultivate a deep and strong friendship, we have to spend time with the one we love in order to talk together and to listen to one another. It is the same in our relationship with God. As we spend time together with him, we learn to know him better and to appreciate him more. As we begin to confide in him more fully, our planned time of prayer turns spontaneously into a period of deep intimacy.

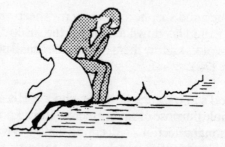

Knowing God as he really is – what a tremendous motivation to pray! What a privilege it is to be with him, to be able to speak to him and to listen to him! I am weak, but he is strong; my days are limited, but he is eternal; I am a sinner, but he is holy . . . My desire to pray springs essentially from who God is.

In Matthew 6:1–18, Jesus speaks six times about his Father rewarding those who fast, pray and give secretly.

What is the nature of this reward which results from spending time in the presence of God?

Listen to these extraordinary words pronounced by Charles Spurgeon (when only twenty years of age!) concerning the way in which God rewards those who take time to come to know him:

'Would you lose your sorrow? Would you drown your cares? Then go, plunge yourself in the Godhead's deepest sea; be lost in his immensity, and you shall come forth as from a couch of rest, refreshed and invigorated.

'I know of nothing which can so comfort the soul; so calm the swelling billows of sorrow and grief; so speak peace to the winds of trial, as a devout musing on the subject of the Godhead. It is to that subject that I invite you this morning...'

Personally, I must admit that I have never found it easy to begin a time of prayer and fasting. Making the decision has often, if not always, been a battle.

However, I can testify that those times spent, secretly, alone with God and his Word have been memorable occasions that I have never regretted.

In God's presence, we discover deep peace and joy, consolation and a liberating power. God's real work in us begins when he touches us deeply and enables us to receive his forgiveness. Oh! How good it is to be able to come close to God!

How should we fast?

Not like the hypocrites who fast only to be seen and admired, but with the right attitude of heart, in genuine humility and in complete dependence on God. For God sees our hearts, and he is more concerned by our motivations for fasting than by the mere fact of our going through the motions.

Fasting is an attitude of the body, the mind and the soul. Since salvation includes our body, mind and soul, it is important that all three should be engaged in prayer.

Jesus teaches us that, fundamentally, fasting is more than simply abstaining from food. Fasting means showing God our real values: it is going without something good with a view to something even better: an intimate relationship with God!

The practical lesson for us:

In Matthew 21:12–17, Jesus becomes angry. For what reason? Because those going to the temple have got their values all wrong. Their business interests have taken the place of the presence of God. Jesus overturns their tables – and by so doing overturns their values: 'My house will be called a house of prayer, but you are making it a den of robbers .'

What are your priorities? What are your values? Can you truly say that your relationship with God comes before watching television, reading for pleasure, making plans for the future, the state of you bank account, and even your activities in the church . . . ? Fasting means finding time to show God that he really does have the first place in our lives.

Now, perhaps it would do us good to miss a meal – or to go without something else which is beginning to occupy too much time and place in our lives – in order to spend time in the presence of God, to talk over our priorities with him so that he can sort them into the right order for us.

A practical suggestion: During your time of prayer and fasting, take a sheet of paper and write down your priorities.

Let us summarize what we have just seen concerning the principles laid down by Jesus and the warnings he gives:

The purpose of fasting is:

1. To come closer to God (not to please others).

2. To express our complete dependence on God and our vital need of his presence and of his Word (our spiritual food).

3. To involve our body, mind and soul in prayer.

Here is an acrostic to help you remember the main points of the teaching of Jesus about fasting:

According to Jesus . . .

Fasting in the right way involves:

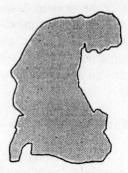

Adjusting one's priorities

Searching one's motives

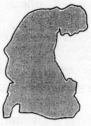

Training one's body

Immersing oneself in the presence of God

Nourishing one's soul with the Word of God

Growing in the knowledge of God

The right way to fast

The teaching of Isaiah

The fast which pleases God – 'the kind of fast I have chosen' (Isa. 58:6).

Fasting that liberates

Isaiah 58:6–7 gives details about the attitude of heart we should have while practising fasting:

'to loose . . . to untie . . . to set free' (Isa. 58:6).

These words speak of a liberation from what hinders, binds and enslaves us.

The apostle expresses the same idea when he writes to the Corinthians:

'I must not be a slave of anything' (1 Co. 6:12).

The practical lesson for us:

We can practise fasting in order to ask God to free us from a bad habit, to liberate us from some vice, in other words to ask God to 'operate' on us at a deep level in a particular area of our life.

Our so-called private life, the thoughts that pass through our minds are important in God's eyes. Are we harbouring resentment or jealousy against someone? Have we a spirit of bitterness?

Are we addicted to any substance or drink (coffee, tea, alcohol) or habit that has a grip on us? Do we do certain things with our body that do not glorify God? Do we read books or watch films that poison our mind?

'Fasting helps us keep our balance in life. How easily we begin to allow non-essentials to take precedence in our lives. How quickly we crave things we do not need until we are enslaved by them. Paul writes, "All things are lawful for me, but I will not be enslaved by anything" (1 Co. 6:12). Our human cravings and desires are like rivers that tend to overflow their banks; fasting helps keep them in their proper channels. "I pummel my body and subdue it," says Paul (1 Co. 9:27). Likewise, David writes, "I afflicted myself with fasting" (Ps. 35:13). This is not excessive asceticism; it is discipline and discipline brings freedom.'[11]

Can we say: 'I am free: no passion or habit dominates me. I am a clean vessel – available to be used by God to channel his blessing to others!'

We can practise fasting alone, but we can also ask a friend to pray with us. We can share with him or her the area in which we are tempted, confess our helplessness, and implore God to work in our life.

Fasting that changes our attitude to others

'Share your food with the hungry' (v. 7).

The word 'share' expresses the idea of generosity and kindness to those around us, the fruit of love and of grace. The opposite of sharing is selfishness, self-centredness and individualism.

In Isaiah 58:7, fasting is accompanied by an attitude of sharing with others, of hospitality ('to provide the poor wanderer with shelter') and of compassion ('when you see the naked, . . . clothe him').

The right kind of fasting is to be available before God, with the right inner spirit (submission, obedience) but also with an attitude of mercy and of compassion towards others expressed in a practical way.

No! says Isaiah, fasting is not a way of forcing God to act in the way you want! Instead, it means offering yourself to God and seeking to correct wrong attitudes and actions in your life.

Let us remind ourselves again that prayer and fasting is not a way of getting what we want but of becoming what God wants us to be. Dr Alexis Carrel, who won the Nobel prize for medicine in 1912, expresses this thought with beautiful imagery: 'In prayer, one offers oneself to God like the canvas before the painter or the marble before the sculptor.'[12]

Here then are Isaiah's answers to the question: What is the purpose of fasting? We fast in order to examine whether our attitudes are pleasing to God. This change of attitude towards God brings about a change in our attitude towards others – sharing, hospitality, compassion.

The practical lesson for us:

Let's practise fasting in order to see our attitudes transformed. Let's ask God to intervene in our life in order to change our selfish indifference towards others into genuine love and compassion, our greed into generosity.

The blessings that accompany the kind of fasting God approves (Isa. 58:6–14)

After setting out the right and the wrong ways to fast, Isaiah speaks of the blessings associated with the kind of fasting that pleases God:

v. 8 'Your light will break forth like the dawn'

A person who practises fasting in the way God wishes will be 'radiant' – reflecting the presence and the glory of the Lord. When Moses had spent forty days and forty nights in the presence of the Lord, 'his face was radiant' – though he himself was unaware of it (Ex. 34:29).

I knew a man about whom someone used to say that 'he carried about with him a square yard of holiness'! My grandmother, a real woman of prayer, was radiant with the presence of the Lord.

'Those who look to him are radiant' (Ps. 34:5).

v. 8 'Your healing will quickly appear'

Illness is often (though not always) provoked by wrong attitudes such as hate, desire for revenge, bitterness, the refusal to forgive, etc. God wants to work deeply in our lives to transform us and to restore us.

v. 8 'Your righteousness will go before you'

v. 8 'The glory of the Lord will be your rear guard'

God will honour us with his presence and assures us of his protection.

'The Lord will go before you, the God of Israel will be your rear guard' (Isa. 52:12).

v. 9 'Then you will call, and the Lord will answer'

David prays because he knows that God answers: 'I call on you, O God, for you will answer me' (Ps. 17:6).

Isaiah has the same certainty: 'As soon as he hears, he will answer' (Isa. 30:19).

In another passage, Isaiah goes even further: 'Before they call I will answer, while they are still speaking I will hear' (Isa. 65:24).

What an encouragement to pray!

v. 10 'Your light will rise in the darkness'

Jesus, himself the true light of the world, tells us: 'You are the world's light . . . Let your light shine . . . in the sight of men' (Mt. 5:14, 16).

What a privilege to be a little light guiding those around us towards God!

v. 11 'The Lord will guide you always'

In good times and bad times, God promises to be with us and to be our guide.

'The Lord is my shepherd, I shall not be in want. He makes me to lie down in green pastures, he leads me beside quiet waters' (Ps. 23:1–2).

'Even though I walk through the valley of the shadow of death, I will fear no evil, for you are with me' (Ps. 23:4).

'When you pass through the waters, I will be with you' (Isa. 43:2).

v. 11 'He will satisfy your needs in a sun-scorched land and will strengthen your frame. You will be like a well-watered garden, like a spring whose waters never fail.'

How to fast in the right way:

– Have the right attitude (Isa. 58:6).

– Know what the Bible teaches (Mt. 6:1–17).

– Fast for the right reasons (Zec. 7:5).

– Always devote time to secret prayer while fasting, and have the right attitude towards God and others (Mt. 6:18).

– Have a balanced view of fasting, avoiding over-emphasis on the subject (Col. 2:23).

A summary of the Bible's teaching on fasting

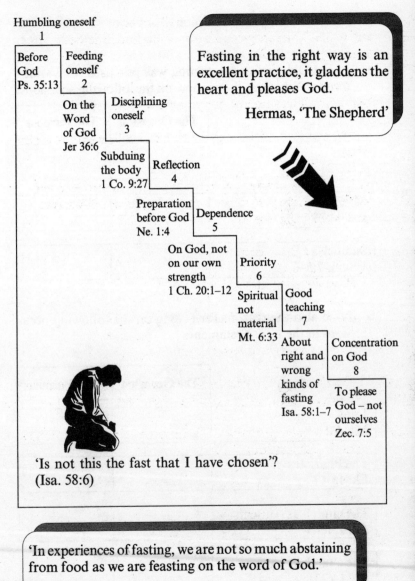

Humbling oneself
1

Before God
Ps. 35:13

Feeding oneself
2

On the Word of God
Jer 36:6

Disciplining oneself
3

Subduing the body
1 Co. 9:27

Reflection
4

Preparation before God
Ne. 1:4

Dependence
5

On God, not on our own strength
1 Ch. 20:1–12

Priority
6

Spiritual not material
Mt. 6:33

Good teaching
7

About right and wrong kinds of fasting
Isa. 58:1–7

Concentration on God
8

To please God – not ourselves
Zec. 7:5

Fasting in the right way is an excellent practice, it gladdens the heart and pleases God.

Hermas, 'The Shepherd'

'Is not this the fast that I have chosen'?
(Isa. 58:6)

'In experiences of fasting, we are not so much abstaining from food as we are feasting on the word of God.'

Richard Foster

5. Questions for further reflection

a. In the Old Testament, fasting was practised for various reasons. What was the purpose on the following occasions:

	The Occasion	The Purpose
Ahab 1 Ki. 21:27		
Moses Ex. 34:28		
Samuel 1 Sam. 7:5–6		

b. Note also the reasons for fasting on the following occasions in the New Testament:

	The Occasion	The Purpose
Jesus Mt. 4:2		
The Pharisees Lk. 18:12		
The church at Antioch Ac. 13:2–3		
The church at Lystra Ac. 14:23		

c. Four basic truths about fasting in the Bible:

– **Fasting is always accompanied by prayer**

Why is it important that we always pray when we fast?

_____

– In what state of mind did Jehoshaphat and Nehemiah fast and pray?

Jehoshaphat (2 Ch. 20:3): _____

Nehemiah (Ne. 1:4): _____

– **Fasting is a gesture of self-humbling**

– What does 'to humble oneself' mean?

_____

– **Fasting is a gesture of solidarity**

– Why is it important to add a practical gesture to our fasting and praying?

_____

– In what way can we give practical expression to our solidarity and compassion?

• To whom could we offer a meal? _____

• To whom could we make a visit? _____

- To whom could we make a gift? _____

- To what person in need could we send the money saved by going without a meal or part of a meal? _____

- Any other practical suggestions? _____

_____

_____

d. Summarize in your own words the gist of the teaching on fasting given by Jesus in Matthew 6:1–18.

_____

_____

e. Try to complete the acrostic using the word 'fasting'.

F _____

A _____

S _____

T _____

I _____

N _____

G _____

The wrong way to fast

f.   Re-read Isaiah 58:1–5? What kind of fasting was God not
     pleased with?

_____

_____

g.   Re-read Zechariah 7. Why did Zechariah reprimand the
     people of Judah?

_____

_____

h.   Why did God, speaking by Jeremiah, say: 'Although they
     fast, I will not listen to their cry' (Jer. 14:12)?

_____

_____

i.   Pages 44 to 53 list the biblical passages which mention
     fasting. The people mentioned on page 94 all practised
     fasting individually or with others. Why was God not
     pleased with their fasting?

_____

_____

> The wrong way to fast according to the Bible

Who?	Passage	Why was their fasting not pleasing to God?
Saul	1 Sam. 14:24–30	
Jezebel	1 Ki. 21:9	
Judah	Zec 7:5	
Pharisees	Lk. 18:12	

Reflection

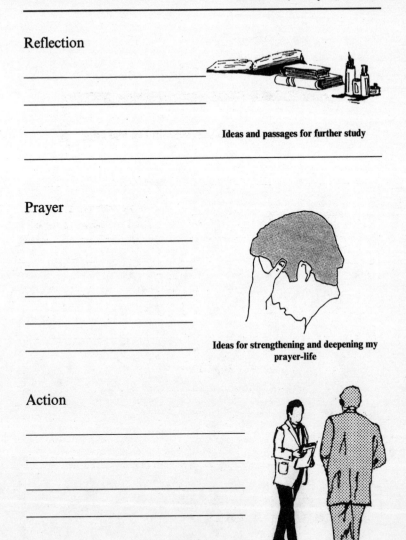

Ideas and passages for further study

Prayer

Ideas for strengthening and deepening my prayer-life

Action

Ideas to put into practice

CHAPTER 3   BIBLICAL EXAMPLES

1. Personal Fasting

A. In the Old Testament
B. In the New Testament

2. Group Fasting

A. In the Old Testament
B. In the New Testament

3. Questions for further reflection

> *I humbled myself with fasting*
>
> *Psalm 35:13*

1. Personal Fasting

A. In the Old Testament

Moses

'Moses was there with the Lord forty days and forty nights without eating bread or drinking water. And he wrote on the tablets the words of the covenant – the Ten Commandments' (Ex. 34:28).

Moses is available for God. He spends time with God. Equally important is his attitude in the presence of God – an attitude of humility, of submission, of dependence and of renunciation.

Moses receives spiritual food for the people from the Lord: 'He wrote on the tablets the words of the covenant – the Ten Commandments' (Ex. 34:28).

This Word of God will instruct, nourish and protect the people down through the centuries. Their devotion to this Word will prompt them to worship and protect them from idolatry (Ex. 20:5).

Moses is surrounded by the presence of God.

'His face was radiant because he had spoken with the Lord' (Ex. 34:29).

Three times the text notes that Moses' face was radiant (vv. 29, 30, 35). Moses was so radiant after being with God that the people were afraid to approach him.

Fasting in order to be wholly available for God

If I fast personally, I do so in order to set aside quality time to spend with God.

Some time ago, I accidentally arranged to meet with two different persons on the same day and at the same time. After realizing my mistake, I had to postpone my meeting with John in order to meet Jim. The conversation with Jim did not go at all well. Physically I was present, but I found it difficult to concentrate: all the time I was thinking of my missed appointment with John. I was available to Jim but only in appearance. Outwardly I had time for him, but inwardly I was ill-prepared to listen and understand what he was trying to communicate to me.

It is the same in my relationship with God. When I spend time with him, I am often unable to immerse myself in his presence and to hear his Word because my mind is preoccupied with other things like my plans for this, my worries about the other, and so on.

In his book, *The Psychology of Prayer*, Pablo Martinez eloquently expresses the relation between prayer and availability:

'To pray is to make ourselves available to God so that he can do in us what he has wanted to do for a long time.'

An amusing story

Here is an amusing but instructive story told by Mr Sundar Krishnan at a missionary conference.[13]

'One day an explorer was preparing to encounter an isolated tribe in the virgin forest. This would require several days' march through the impenetrable equatorial jungle, so he hired the services of about twenty native porters to carry his equipment. He reckoned that the journey would take about ten days. At the end of the first day, he was pleasantly surprised when his porters covered about twice the expected distance.

'However, the next day he had a further surprise: none of the porters would make a move. He brought them together and asked them to start walking. They stoutly refused. When he asked them the reason for their attitude, their reply astonished him: "We walked much too quickly yesterday: our souls could not keep up with our bodies. So we have to stop here until they do!" '

Perhaps we smile at this story, but we would do well to think about it carefully. The pace of life in our western civilization is in the process of detaching us from our souls – with the result that many people do not even remember they have one, much less that they need to take care of it? As Christians, we are not immune to this stress – it just invades the spiritual realm as well. In no time at all our diary fills up with all sorts of activities and meetings. Unable to keep pace with our outward occupations, we gradually succumb to an inward emptiness. No time is left for prayer and meditation, nor even to think before we act. Whenever a problem arises, we immediately invent a solution and draw up an action plan. This is the way businesses have to operate in order to battle against their competitors. Have we not all been influenced by their example?

We need to take care of our souls! In the midst of our activities, let us be careful not to leave our souls behind lest we create a breach which the enemy of our souls will exploit. When king David began to experience this inner emptiness, he expressed it in terms of soul thirst: 'O God, you are my God, earnestly I seek you; my soul thirsts for you, my body longs for you in a dry and weary land where there is no water. I have seen you in the sanctuary and beheld your power and your glory' (Ps. 63:1–2). So it is in God's sanctuary – in his presence – that our soul can catch up with our body.'

Let's take time to be available for God!

When we make a telephone call, we sometimes hear the words: 'The line is busy, please call later.' In other words, the line is not available. At other times, my correspondent's line is available but another voice informs me that my correspondent, though present, is not available.

In other words, the person is there but occupied with more important things.

Listen to this beautiful prayer composed by the French scientist, and writer, Blaise Pascal. It expresses an attitude of tranquillity, of confidence and total submission to God:

'Only you know what is good for me. Therefore give to me, or take from me, as you think best. Bend my will to yours. May I accept with humble and perfect submission and with holy confidence the way you order my life by your eternal providence. May I accept in the same way everything that comes to me from you. Through Jesus Christ our Lord. Amen.'[14]

The lesson for us:

Here is some practical advice about ways to help create this availability, this inward tranquillity, during your time of prayer and fasting:

Plan your fast: Try to plan ahead for your time of prayer and fasting (whether personal or collective) by setting aside the necessary time in your diary.

Find a quiet place: In our twentieth century, silence is golden. If you cannot find a quiet place where you live, remember that there are places in the country run by Christians where one can spend time in quiet meditation.

Choose the right time: If you decide to fast at home, then fast at a time when you can be undisturbed – for example, the day when the children eat at the canteen, or when you husband is away on business, etc. Your fast ought not to pose problems for those who live with you.

Make a list of your preoccupations: Whenever I begin a fast, I take a sheet of paper and write down everything I have on my mind at the time. This gives me a number of topics to pray about.

Read the Bible: During a fast, we should be feeding on the Word of God. I encourage you to converse with God by alternating prayer and reading the Bible.

Here are some suggestions for suitable passages to read while fasting.

Ps. 63	'My soul thirsts for you.'
Ps. 51	'Wash me and I will be whiter than snow.'
Ps. 18	'I love you, O Lord, my strength, my fortress and my deliverer.'
Ps. 116	'I love the Lord, for he heard my voice.'
Ps. 119:33–40	'Teach me . . . Turn me . . . Give me understanding.'
Ps. 23	'The Lord is my shepherd . . . I will fear no evil.'
Ps. 86	'Bring joy to your servant.'
Ps. 16	'You will fill me with joy in your presence.'

A selection of psalms reflecting different attributes of God:

Ps. 29	God is almighty.
Ps. 19	God is glorious.
Ps. 139	God knows my past, my present and my future. His knowledge is infinite.
Ps. 136	God's love endures for ever.
Ps. 104	The Creator watches over his creation.
Ps. 103	God is compassionate and gracious, and willing to forgive.
Ps. 93	God reigns. He is robed in majesty.
Ps. 92	God's works are great, his thoughts are profound.
Ps. 96	The Lord is king: let all the universe praise him!
Ps. 97	The great God of the universe.

David: fasting after defeat

'They mourned and wept and fasted till evening for Saul and his son Jonathan and for the army of the Lord and the house of Israel, because they had fallen by the sword' (2 Sam. 1:12).

On this occasion, David and his friends fasted because they had been defeated. Saul, the Lord's anointed, had just died and the people of Israel had suffered a crushing defeat at the hands of the enemy (1 Sam. 31:1–13).

God often permits his people to be defeated on account of sin. Sin in our personal life or in the life of the church grieves the Holy Spirit. By fasting and prayer we can repent, expressing to God our own grief and allowing him to search our hearts.

'Search me, O God, and know my heart; test me and know my anxious thoughts. See if there is any offensive way in me, and lead me in the way everlasting' (Ps. 139:23–24).

Saul's valiant men: fasting in sorrow

'Then they took their bones and buried them under a tamarisk tree at Jabesh, and they fasted seven days' (1 Sam. 31:13).

The death of someone close to us reminds us that we are not immortal and that one day it will be our turn to stand before God and to give an account of our life (Ro. 14:12). In such circumstances, time set apart for prayer and fasting can enable us to reorder our priorities and to make decisions with a view to investing our lives for eternity.

Samuel, Nehemiah: fasting to ask forgiveness

In the lives of Samuel, Saul, David, Ahab, Ezra and Nehemiah confession was often accompanied by fasting.

Fasting in this context is an outward sign of inward sorrow. Samuel and Nehemiah bring the people together in order to confront them with their sin. Displaying great courage and refusing to compromise, they expose sin and require the people to confess their faults, to repent and to reform their lives. Nehemiah does not consider such fasting in a negative way but as positive, constructive 'celebration' leading to freedom and blessing (Ne. 9:1).

Repentance is the way to pass from darkness to light (Ro. 10:9), to have our sins wiped out and to experience a time of renewal (Ac. 3:19). To hate sin and to break off sinning is a vital part of sanctification. Augustine taught that 'The confession of evil deeds is the beginning of good deeds.'

The practical lesson for us:

This break with sin is possible as a result of the work of Jesus on the cross. So the cross must be central in our prayers and in our thoughts and lives.

Why not set aside a definite period (a morning or a whole day) in order to spend time in the presence of God? We could nourish our fast on a good number of passages from the Bible and examine ourselves in the mirror of God's Word.

Ezra and Nehemiah: fasting to express their solidarity

Ezra and Nehemiah feel totally at one with the people of God. When the people suffer, they suffer with them; when the people sin, they are grieved and intercede for them.

'Ezra ate no food and drank no water, because he continued to mourn over the unfaithfulness of the exiles' (Ezr. 10:6).

'When I heard these things, I sat down and wept. For some days I mourned and fasted and prayed before the God of heaven' (Ne. 1:4).

The people of God were suffering in captivity. The little 'remnant' remaining in Jerusalem were living in great poverty. The walls of the city were in ruins and its gates had been burned down. Why had all this happened? Because of the people of Judah's sin (2 Ki. 21:1–10; 24:3).

The practical lesson for us:

In our contemporary world, sin is rife: violence, corruption, immorality, war, racism, occult practices, and so on. We know that 'the heart is deceitful above all things and beyond cure' (Jer. 17.9). Moses, David, Isaiah, Josiah, Jehoshaphat, Ezra, Nehemiah and Jeremiah in the Old Testament, like Jesus and Paul in the New Testament, often prayed and even wept on account of the sins of their generation.

At a time of prayer and fasting, we too can express our sorrow at the way things are – and ask God to help people understand that the heart of the problem does not lie in the way society is organized but in their own rebellion against God. We can pray that there will be true repentance and a real turning to God and to his Word.

Daniel: fasting in order to pray more fervently

'So I turned to the Lord God and pleaded with him in prayer and petition, in fasting, and in sackcloth and ashes' (Da. 9:3).

Daniel devotes himself wholly to prayer. Following his fast (Da. 9:22), God teaches him, opening his intelligence and giving him a vision of his glory (Da. 10:10).

In order to pray well, we need time, concentration, quietness and determination. Just as the carpenter, using a little oil, sharpens the blade of his plane on a stone, so the Christian, anointed by the Holy Spirit, can 'sharpen' prayer by fasting.

The practical lesson for us:

For me prayer is always a battle. I often lack the spiritual energy to intercede with warmth and depth, with boldness and fervour. Nonetheless my times of fasting and prayer are always occasions when in a unique way I can realize the presence of God in my life, express to him my hunger and thirst for his presence and humble myself before him. They are times when I am able to concentrate more readily and be particularly aware of the spiritual realm. In this particular contact with God, he can give me insight and discernment concerning my personal life, my family life, my church life and my service for him.

B. In the New Testament

Jesus

'Then Jesus was led by the Spirit into the desert, to be tempted by the devil. After a fast of forty days and nights he was very hungry' (Mt. 4:1–2).

The prolonged fasting practised on this occasion by Jesus was exceptional and reminds us of Moses. Just as Moses delivered his people out of slavery, so Jesus came to liberate us from sin. Moses was the mediator between God and the people; Jesus is our mediator with the Father (1 Ti. 2:5). Moses received God's Word for the people; Jesus is the Word of God (Jn. 1:1).

We have already mentioned the prolonged fasting practiced by Jesus. In his '*Institutes of the Christian Religion*', Calvin commented:

'It is plain that Christ did not fast to set an example to others, but, by thus commencing the preaching of the Gospel, meant to prove that his doctrine was not of men, but had come from heaven.'

Anna, the prophetess

Lk. 2:37 'She spent her whole life in the temple and worshipped God night and day, with fastings and prayers.'

For Anna, fasting was a way of serving God and expressing her love for him.

Paul

Ac. 9:9 Immediately after his conversion, he went three days without food and drink.

2 Co. 6:5 While writing about his suffering and trials, he also mentions fasting.

2 Co. 11:27 Here he mentions having frequently experienced 'hunger and thirst' and 'doing without meals'.

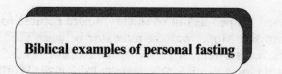

Biblical examples of personal fasting

Note briefly the motivation of the following Bible characters:

Moses
Ex. 34:28
Intimacy and availability in God's presence in order to receive God's Word to feed the people.

Ezra
Ezr. 10:6
Sorrow on account of Israel's sin.

Nehemiah
Ne. 1:4–10
Nehemiah stops, weeps, fasts and prays before going into action. He thought the situation through in God's presence.

David
Ps. 35:13
David fasts on account of opposition and oppression.

Jonathan
1 Sam. 20:34
Jonathan is saddened by the attitude of Saul, his father.

Ahab 1 Ki. 21:29	Ahab humbles himself before God on account of his sin.
Esther Est. 4:10–17	Esther expresses her solidarity with her people when their very existence is threatened.
Isaiah Isa. 58:7	God states that the true meaning of fasting is to have the right attitude towards God (repentance), towards others (compassion) and towards oneself (discipline).
Daniel Da. 9:3	Daniel humbles himself before God and presents his petitions. God answers him.
Jesus Mt. 4:1–2	Before proclaiming the whole counsel of God, Jesus withdraws to a quiet place to fast and pray, giving physical expression to the thought that 'Man shall not live by bread alone, but by every word that proceeds from the mouth of God.'
Anna Lk. 2.37	Anna expresses her devotion to God by prayer and fasting.
Paul Ac. 9:9	Paul fasts following his conversion and the revolution it brought about in his life.

2. Group fasting

A. In the Old Testament

Fasting to humble oneself

The words 'fast' and 'fasting' do not occur in the Hebrew text of the Pentateuch. If we are looking for references to fasting, we must take into account expressions like 'humble your souls' (Lev. 16:29, 31; 23:27; Nu. 29:7). The annual fast was an important date in the Jewish calendar (Ac. 27:9). It was a sacred assembly (Lev. 23:7–8, 23, 35) at which they were to humble themselves before God.

Numbers 29:7–8 mentions that this 'sacred assembly' was to be devoted exclusively to God: 'You must . . . do no work.' This fast was accompanied by voluntary offerings.

During this fast, the Israelites were invited to:

- meet their holy God
- humble themselves before him
- become conscious of their sin
- confess their sins
- implore the purification of all the people

The practical lesson for us:

On several occasions when Hudson Taylor's missionary society was troubled by strained relationships, he called a day of prayer and fasting, and invited all the missionaries to humble themselves before God, confessing their sins of back-biting, bitterness, jealousy and negative attitudes. In this way, these faults were swept away and the mission experienced renewed times of blessing and refreshment.

Could we not experience such times in our churches and organizations?

'Now you must repent [change direction] and turn to God so that your sins may be wiped out, that time after time your souls may know the refreshment that comes from the presence of God' (Ac. 3:19).

Fasting in order to seek guidance

'The Moabites and Ammonites with some of the Meunites came to make war on Jehoshaphat . . . Alarmed, Jehoshaphat resolved to inquire of the Lord, and he proclaimed a fast for all Judah' (2 Ch. 20:1,3).

The people of God were being attacked on all sides. At their wit's end 'the people of Judah came together to seek help from the Lord; indeed they came from every town in Judah to seek him' (v 4). And they fasted as they sought to know God's will.

The practical lesson for us:

Sometimes God places us in difficult circumstances in order to draw us closer to him. By fasting, we express our need of God, our desire to seek his face, his help and his deliverance in the midst of the storm.

In every church or missionary society, important decisions have to be taken constantly: appointing elders or deacons, beginning a new activity, starting a daughter church, building

new premises, moving to a different area, raising finance . . .
It is good to pray and fast when making decisions – not with
the idea of automatically obtaining an immediate answer, but
in order to seek God and learn his will.

Fasting in repentance

'On that day they fasted and there they confessed, "We
have sinned against the Lord." ' (1 Sam. 7:6).

Samuel called on all the people to fast in order for them to:

- come together
- pray to the Lord
- confess their sins
- be judged by Samuel
- eradicate sin in all its forms

'The Ninevites believed God. They declared a fast, and all
of them, from the greatest to the least, put on sackcloth' (Jnh.
3:5).

v. 7 The kings decree: 'Do not let any man or beast, herd
or flock, taste anything; do not let them eat or drink. But let
man and beast be covered with sackcloth. Let everyone call
urgently on God. Let them give up their evil ways and their
violence!'

'On the twenty-fourth day of the same month, the Israelites
gathered together, fasting and wearing sackcloth and having
dust on their heads'.

For three hours, they read in the Law of the Lord, and for three more hours, they confessed their sin and worshipped God (Ne. 9:1–3).

The practical lesson for us:

This process of inner cleansing by means of repentance is possible only on account of the work of Jesus on the cross. That is why the cross must be central in our prayers, our thoughts and our lives. Confessing our sins must be a daily discipline in our personal lives and in the life of our church. Even the preacher cannot bring his message effectively and in power unless he has himself repented and been cleansed of his sins through the blood of Christ. The confession of sin has the double effect of closing the devil's mouth and of opening up a spring of spiritual refreshment. In our churches we need to learn to fear God and to hate sin in all its forms. Sin is anything that takes the place of God in our lives. Let us be like Nehemiah who put Israel's house in order by dealing radically with sin and experience inner cleansing (Ne. 9:1–38).

Let us be careful, however! We should not disclose to everyone in the church sins which do not concern them all. Some sins are committed only against God, and some are committed only against certain people. If in doubt, we should seek the advice of a pastor or elder.

Confessing our faults to another person helps to keep us humble (Jas. 5:16).

'By confessing our sins in prayer, we express to God our incapacity to purify our own hearts' (Ps. 51:1–19).[15]

Fasting in order to remember

After the Exile, four fasts were introduced into the Jewish calendar. In Zechariah 8:19 the prophet mentions these four fasts which were reminders of important but sad events in the history of Israel:

Fourth month:
- A great famine at Jerusalem (Jer. 52:6).
- Israel's disobedience in the matter of the golden calf (Ex. 20).
- Manasseh's placing an idol in the house of God (2 Ch.33:7).

Fifth month:
- The destruction of the Temple (Zec.7:3).

Seventh month:
- The death of Gedaliah, appointed governor of Judah by the king of Babylon and assassinated by Ishmael (Jer. 41:2).

Tenth month:
- In memory of the siege of Jerusalem by Nebuchadnezzar (Jer. 52:12–13).

According to Zechariah, for the people of Judah these fast-days became joyful and glad occasions and happy festivals.

Fasting before beginning an important task

'I proclaimed a fast, so that we might humble ourselves before our God and ask him for a safe journey . . .' Ezra implores the protection of God for himself and for the people before leaving for Jerusalem where they will rebuild the Temple (Ezr. 8:21).

Note that several years later, when the walls of the city had been rebuilt, 'all the people [of God] assembled as one man' (Ne. 8:1). Thus Ezra was God's instrument for bringing revival to the people and for preserving it amongst them. This revival was one of the greatest spiritual awakenings in the entire history of Israel.

The practical lesson for us:

Before beginning a new project, leaving on a journey, moving house, or starting a new job, taking a new direction in life, let us learn to stop and ask God to give us wisdom, protection and guidance.

Fasting in order to listen to God and his Word

'The Israelites gathered together, fasting and wearing sackcloth . . . They stood where they were and read from the Book of the Law of the Lord their God for a quarter of the day' (Ne. 9:1,3).

Our fast will be biblical only if we feast on the delicious bread of Holy Scripture. The reading of God's Word is the spark that will kindle our heart as we pray. The Word will make our fast appetising and give direction to our prayer – so that it becomes a dialogue with God. Without the Word, prayer degenerates into sheer mysticism; without prayer, reading the Word degenerates into mere intellectualism. Fasting and prayer serve to detach ourselves deliberately from the practical preoccupations which usually encumber our mind. They create in our spirit a fertile soil in which the seed of the Word of God can fall and take root.

The practical lesson for us:

Jeremiah states what we should do when we fast:

'Go to the house of the Lord on a day of fasting and read to the people from the scroll the words of the Lord that you wrote as I dictated. Read them to all the people of Judah who come in from their towns' (Jer. 36:6).

Throughout their history, the people of Israel often set aside a solid block of time – a morning or a whole day or several days – in order to fast, to pray and to read or hear the Word of God. What a privilege to take time to listen to the Word of God!

From time to time we too should break with the many things that encumber our minds by leaving aside our discussions, consultations, committees and meetings devoted to administration in order to steep ourselves in the Word of God.

Psalm 119 makes excellent reading during a fast. It expresses our thirst for God's Word, our burning desire to allow it to penetrate deeply into our heart. Note the different requests that figure in this prayer:

'Teach me, O Lord, to follow your decrees, then I will keep them to the end. Give me understanding, and I will keep your law and obey it with all my heart. Direct me in the path of your commands; for there I find delight. Turn my heart towards your statutes and not toward selfish gain. Turn my eyes away from worthless things; preserve my life according to your word.

Fulfil your promise to your servant, so that you may be feared. Take away the disgrace I dread, for your laws are good. How I long for your precepts! Preserve my life in your righteousness!' (Ps. 119:33–40).

Reading this psalm can enrich our time of fasting and help us appreciate the value of the Word of God which is given to us to obey.

Here are three beautiful prayers which I have often used before – and sometimes after – my reading of the Scriptures:

O God, inexhaustible source of all good,
I praise you for the gifts of your love.
Give me grace to listen to your Word
with attention and respect, with a sincere desire
to believe its promises and to obey its commands.
Engrave your Word,
not only in my mind
but also in my heart,
and change me by your Spirit
into the image of your Son
through contemplating your truth
in the clear mirror of your Gospel.
Amen.

O Lord, your Word is to us, your creatures,
the seed of life, the yeast of the Kingdom,
the germ of hope.
Dispose my heart and mind to receive
your Word with simplicity and with joy.
May your Word enable me to bear
the good fruit that you look for in my life.
Through Jesus Christ our Lord.
Amen.

As a child receives bread
as a bird receives the grain
as a friend receives a friend
as the night receives the dawn
and the sunshine
as the soil receives the seed
as the sap rises in the branches
and bears fruit
grant me, O Lord,
to receive your Word.
Amen.

(Reformed Church of France, used by permission)

B. In the New Testament

The disciples of John the Baptist – fasting frequently

'John's disciples are always fasting and praying' (Lk. 5:33).

The leaders of the church at Antioch – fasting before sending missionaries

'While they were worshipping the Lord and fasting, the Holy Spirit spoke to them, saying, "Set Barnabas and Saul apart for me for a task to which I have called them" ' (Ac. 13:2).

The church at Antioch was enriched by the presence of several teachers, prophets . . . and missionaries. It was while they fasted that Barnabas and Saul were marked out by the Holy Spirit.

Jesus instructs us to pray to the Lord of the harvest to send out workers (Mt. 9:38). The church at Antioch prays, fasts and sends out a small team of missionaries who will in turn plant other churches. What a team they were!

The practical lesson for us:

I know a church in France that regularly meets to fast and pray that God will send out workers all over the world. The money saved on the meal is sent to a missionary society. Let us take seriously our responsibility not only to support missionary work but also to encourage our church to pray to the Lord of the harvest to send workers into his harvest.

Paul and Barnabas – Fasting before choosing church elders

After starting churches at Lystra, Iconium and Antioch, Paul and Barnabas 'appointed elders for them in each church, and with prayer and fasting commended them to the Lord in whom they had believed' (Ac. 14:23).

The practical lesson for us:

We can encourage the church to pray and fast before appointing elders. The time set aside by the whole church can be used for reflection and Bible study on the spiritual and moral qualifications required to be an elder. All this must be undertaken without haste and with great care.

The Jews: fasting before confronting sin

'. . . by now it was after the Fast' (Ac. 27:9, NIV).

This was the annual fast on the Day of Atonement prescribed in Leviticus 16:29–31. This 'sacred assembly' was held at the end of September. It appears that this annual fast was still observed by the Jews in New Testament times.

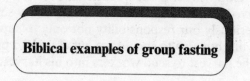

Biblical examples of group fasting

Briefly note the motivation for fasting of the groups of persons mentioned in the following passages:

Occasion	Text	Motivation
Annual fast	Lev. 16:19–34	Humbling themselves before God
War	Jdg. 20:26–28	Seeking guidance
National fast	1 Sam. 7:6	Confessing sin
Invasion	2 Ch. 20:3–4	Seeking the Lord

Occasion	Text	Motivation
Before returning from Exile	Ezr. 8:21	Asking for protection
During the Exile	Isa. 58:6–7	A change of attitude towards God and others
After returning from Exile	Ne. 9:1–3	Listening to God's Word
Disaster	Joel 2:12	Returning to God
Revival at Nineveh	Jnh. 3:5	Turning from evil ways
Prophetic fasting	Zec. 8:19	Gratitude to God
Sending missionaries	Ac. 14:2	Before appointing and sending Paul and Barnabas
Appointing elders	Ac 14:23	After appointing elders in several churches

3. **Questions for further reflection**

A. **Personal fasting**

a. In what way was Moses' fast exceptional?

Exodus 34:28–35 _____

_____

_____

_____

_____

_____

b. Nehemiah's fast was accompanied by three other actions. What were they?

Nehemiah 1:4 _____

_____

_____

_____

_____

c. Nehemiah's fast was followed by a beautiful prayer (Ne. 1:5–11). Note the different attributes of God mentioned in this prayer:

_____

_____

_____

_____

d. What prevents us from spending quality time with God?

_____

_____

_____

_____

e. What can we do to overcome these obstacles?

_____

_____

_____

_____

B. Group fasting

According to the following passages, what is the purpose of group fasting?

a. 2 Chronicles 20:1–4 _____

_____

b. 1 Samuel 7:3–8 _____

_____

c. Joel 2:15–17 _____

_____

d. Acts 13:3–4 _____

_____

e. Acts 14:21–23 _____

_____

Reflection

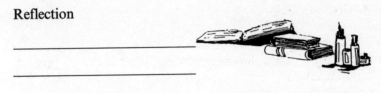

_____

_____

_____

Ideas and passages for further study

_____

Prayer

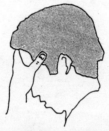

_____

_____

_____

_____

_____

**Ideas for strengthening and deepening my
prayer-life**

Action

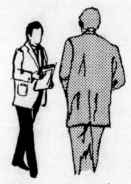

_____

_____

_____

_____

_____

Ideas to put into practice

CHAPTER 4   HOW TO FAST – PERSONALLY AND COLLECTIVELY

1. In what circumstances should we fast?

2. What should we do before, during and after fasting?

3. Questions for further reflection.

> *Fasting is a useless and even dangerous remedy for one who is ignorant of why and how to fast.*
>
> *John Chrysostom*

1. In what circumstances should we fast?

Our fast should always be centred on God. We should fast to please God, not ourselves (Zec. 7:5).

'God himself becomes much more important than our request. This is the deepest and most enriching aspect of prayer,' writes Oswald Chambers. 'The meaning of prayer is holding on to God rather than to the answer . . . Communion with God is what the soul needs more than anything else . . . When amidst all his gifts we find him, we find all.'[16]

If we do not fast to please God, then we have failed. John Wesley wrote: 'Let us fast unto the Lord, keeping our eyes fixed on him alone.' May our motivation be the desire to please our Father in heaven. In this way we will be preserved from appreciating the gifts more than the Giver. Once the main object and motivation for fasting are clear in our minds, we are free to have other motivations for fasting in addition.

Here are some good reasons for fasting personally or collectively:

Intimacy with God: We want to spend more time with God.

Earnestness: To show God we are in earnest.
To intercede with all our heart.
To express sorrow after sinning.

Guidance and help: To ask God for guidance before making a major decision (about our career, marriage, an expensive purchase, etc).
To ask God's help at a difficult time.

Solidarity: To show God our rejection of individualism and our desire to share our joys and suffering within our group (1 Co.12:26).

Liberty: To show God that we are not slaves to food (Lk. 21:34).

Humility: To confess our faults. By fasting and prayer, we crucify our sinful nature with its desires and we ask Jesus to purify us.

Listening to God: To enable us to listen to God and to his Word.

2. What should we do before, during and after fasting?

A few days before fasting

* Read the Bible passages about fasting, then try to identify your reason and motivation for fasting. Pray about it.

* Decide on a date and inform your family or other people with whom you live or work.

* Postpone any appointments or activities originally planned at this time.

* If your fasting is likely to pose problems for them, it would be better to postpone it until you can fast alone.

* Choose a book of the Bible to read or study during your fast. (See the suggested selection of psalms on pages 103–104.)

* Prepare two or three books to read during your fast. I can suggest a few that I have already 'relished' and enjoyed at such times:

  – *From Now On*, R. Shallis (STL)
  – *Knowing God*, J I Packer (Hodders)
  – *Power Through Prayer*, E M Bounds (CLC)
  – *Prayer*, Richard Foster (Hodders)
  – *Celebration of Discipline*, R. Foster (Hodders)
  – *No Turning Back*, George Verwer (STL)
  – *Revival*, Martyn Lloyd-Jones (Marshalls)
  – *Strengthening Your Grip*, C.Swindoll (Hodders)
  – *Ordering Your Private World*, George Macdonald, (Highland Books)
  – *52 Meditations and Prayers of Martin Luther* (Concordia)

* 'You should decide how long to continue fasting before you begin. Your body will then know instinctively how much time is available for its purification and renewal and will apportion its strength accordingly.'[17]

* During the previous day or several days, start diminishing the amount of food you eat at each meal.

* Talk about your intentions to a Christian friend who has already practised fasting. Ask him to pray that your time of fasting will glorify God and be a positive experience for you.

* Try to draw up a timetable for the period of fasting. (See pages 140–142 for an example.)

The day before

* Prepare all the things you may need:

  – water, fruit juice, vegetable juice, herbal teas
  – warm clothes
  – hot-water bottle
  – walking shoes
  – Bible, books, notebook
  – music or message cassettes
  – hymn book

* Eat sparingly at midday and in the evening

* Go to bed early.

During your fast

My own experience: What I have noticed about my times of fasting and prayer.

A desire to pray more:

Today I am fasting. I note that during this time, I have greater facility and energy in prayer than at other times. Once I begin, I don't want to stop!

I go out into the country and walk alongside a field of lavender. I speak aloud to God, as I would to a friend. I have with me a hymn book and the Book of Common Prayer of the Church of England. As I walk, I read and sing in order to 'feed' my time of prayer. I am conscious of the presence of God and of the fact that he loves me and is coming to my aid.

There are so many people to intercede for and so many subjects to pray about. However, above all I want to spend time intimately with God – praising him and listening to him.

An awareness of the state of my own heart

While fasting, it is not unusual for all kinds of bad feelings to 'surface' (jealousy, bitterness, fear, anxiety). Is this due to the devil accusing me – or to the Holy Spirit showing me a sin that needs to be confessed? If it is the devil, he will simply accuse me and make me feel discouraged. If it is the Holy Spirit, he will 'put his finger' on a definite occasion where I was at fault and will call on me to repent. I will then read aloud Psalm 51 and ask God to forgive me and to purify me of my sin and to restore the joy of my salvation.

Remember that Jesus himself was attacked by the devil while he fasted for forty days and nights in the desert (Lk. 4:2). When we fast, our body is in a state of weakness, and we ourselves are more vulnerable to temptation. It is possible for the devil to seize this occasion to prowl around us, and to harass and attack us. This is one reason we need to feed on the Word of God while fasting. Then, like Jesus, we can put the adversary to flight using a sharp thrust of our powerful and effective 'sword', the Word of God.

Some practical ideas about how to use your time while fasting

* Write a letter to God during this time.

* Meditate on God and on his attributes and works. The passages listed on pages 103–4 can serve as a basis for meditation. I encourage you to list God's attributes, to define them and to think carefully about each one of them. In the prayer recorded in Nehemiah 9:5–37, an impressive number of divine attributes are mentioned. J. I. Packer's book *Knowing God* has impressed me by its depth. It even brought me to tears as it made me realize the greatness of God's grace and love to a poor sinner like me.

* Go for a walk in the country and contemplate the marvels of God's creation. 'The works of God speak about his invisible perfections to the minds and conscience of mankind: whoever knows how to look can clearly discern in them the reality and the power of God' (Ro. 1:20, paraphrased by A. Kuen).

* Listen to some beautiful music!!

* List all the blessings that God has given you this year. 'Count your blessings – and it will surprise you what the Lord has done!'

* Use this quiet period to study a book or a Bible theme. *How to Study the Bible for Yourself* by T. Lahaye (Harvest House) will prove useful.

* Do a few physical exercises.

* Spend an hour conversing with God – in **A**doration, **C**onfession, **T**hanksgiving and **S**upplication / intercession (= **ACTS**). I encourage you to buy the book *How To Spend an Hour with God* by Dick Eastman (Vida). It is simple, practical and biblical!

* Drink frequently.

* Read the biography of a man or woman of God like Catherine Booth, David Brainerd, Amy Carmichael, James Fraser, George Müller, Murray M'Cheyne, Charles Spurgeon, Hudson Taylor, Suzanne Wesley.

* Write a letter to an old friend thanking him for his help, his example and his faithfulness over the years. As we encourage others, we are encouraged ourselves!

* Meditate on a verse or passage of the Bible. Richard Foster's book *Celebration of Discipline* has a chapter explaining how to meditate and others on how to fast, how to pray, how to read a book and how to study.

* Intercede for the world. Use information gleaned from the newspaper, the television or the radio. *Operation World* (WEC) is a mine of information to help us pray intelligently about every country in the world.

* Have a time of rest and relaxation at least three times during the day. 'Unwind!'

* Write down in a notebook your priorities for the coming months and years.

* Sing a hymn you particularly enjoy.

* Intercede for your family, your church, your town and your county. List your petitions relating to each of them and note an appropriate verse from the Bible.

* Intercession for other Christians must be a priority. Pray for the Christians you know – God's 'instruments' for evangelizing the world!

Use Colossians 1:9–12 as a pattern as you pray that Christians may experience spiritual stability, growth and progress:

verse 9:

a. Fill them with the knowledge of your will:

– Show them what you want them to do today.
– Help them to witness to people lovingly.
– Help them to know what to say and how to answer their questions.

b. Fill them with spiritual wisdom and intelligence:

– Open their eyes to understand your plans.
– Help them see things as you do.
– Show them the reason for their difficulties.
– Help them to learn from difficult circumstances.

verse 10:

c. Enable them to walk in a way worthy of you.

– Help them to be kind and courteous to all.
– Give them all the patience they need.
– May others see Jesus in them today.

d. May they please you in all they do.

– Help them to choose the best for other people.
– Give them an opportunity to serve you today.
– If they have sinned, help them to confess at once.

e. Use their life to produce beautiful fruit:

– Let them meet people who are seeking God.
– Help them to walk in the Spirit.
– Give them compassion for those in need.

f. Help them to grow in knowledge.

– Help them to know you more intimately.
– Make them your devoted servants.
– May they see life as you see it.

verse 11:

g. Give them strength.

– Give them the desire to pray.
– Fill them with a new love for your Word.
– Remind them of past lessons you taught them.

h. Help them to become patient and persevering.

– May each trial leave them stronger than before.
– May they be patient and avoid getting angry.

i. Give them a joyful heart.

– May they find their joy in Jesus.
– Fill them with your love today.
– May they not be discouraged by difficulties.
– Fill them with gratitude for your goodness.

verse 12:

j. May they grow more and more like Jesus.

– Give them compassion for those who suffer.
– May they learn to forgive those who wrong them.
– Make them useful in your service.
– May they be an example to me.

Practical advice for the beginner

How to begin.

Your fast may be short or long:

* missing one meal
* from midday to the following morning
* 24 hours, 35 hours, 48 hours, or even longer

What matters is not so much the length of your fast as your motivation and how much you really want to spend time with God and in his Word.

Here is a suggestion as to how to fast for 24 hours. It does not have to be followed in detail. What matters is taking practical steps to avoid being unoccupied and becoming lethargic. I want to encourage you to spend your time of fasting in doing worthwhile things!

8am–9am   Throw your windows wide open: Do a few physical exercises. Have a good shower. Go for a walk in the garden, in a park or in the country. Pray aloud, thanking God for the beauty of nature: the flowers, the trees, the birds! Take your Bible with you and stop from time to time to read a magnificent verse or two from Psalm 96. For example, verses 11–12: 'Let the heavens rejoice, let the earth be glad; let the sea resound and all that is in it; let the fields be jubilant and everything in them. Then all the trees of the forest will sing for joy.' Interrupt your reading to pray or sing.

9am–10am   Write a brief letter to God. Tell him your hopes, your fears, and above all your reasons for setting aside this time to spend with him. (What we say, we quickly forget, what we write, stays in our mind.)

10am–12.30pm Study time. Re-read Chapter 2 entitled 'Fasting in the Bible', then answer the questions at the end of the chapter.

12.30–2pm   Have a siesta, go for a walk or read a chapter from a book of your choice. (If you do not know what to read, consult the list of suitable books suggested on page 132.)

2pm–3pm   Take time to examine your life in the light of the Word of God and of the Holy Spirit. For example, read aloud Psalm 51, praying after each verse. You could also read Psalm 119:33–40 or Psalm 139:23, 24: 'Search me, O God, and know my heart; test me and know my anxious thoughts. See if there is any offensive way in me, and lead me in the way everlasting.'

3pm–4pm   Unwind! Listen to some beautiful music and – weather permitting – sit for awhile in the sunshine.

4pm–6pm   Write down a list of Bible characters who practised fasting. Re-read Chapter 3 of this book and answer the questions at the end of the chapter.

6pm–7pm	Have a time of prayer for your family, your friends, your church, your town, your country, and other parts of the world. Make lists, note appropriate Bible verses. This will help you to pray with precision.
7pm–8pm	You could use this time to write a letter of encouragement and gratitude to someone who was a great help to you at an important time in your life (a parent, a Sunday School teacher, a youth leader, a pastor or elder . . .).
8pm–10pm	I have made other suggestions on pages 135 to 137. To conclude your day of fasting, I suggest you write down a brief summary of how you spent the day, and of what it has meant to you. It will be prove useful to you on future occasions as well as help you share your experience with other Christians.

Good night!

A brief evaluation:

Why not write down in a little notebook your thoughts about this time of fasting and prayer? Would you say that it helped you to be more available to God? Were God and his Word at the centre of the time you set aside?

If so, why not make a new appointment to spend time with God in prayer and fasting?

3. Questions for further reflection

a. What precautions should one take . . .

* before fasting?

_____

_____

_____

_____

* while fasting?

_____

_____

_____

_____

* after fasting?

_____

_____

_____

_____

b. If you plan to have a day of fasting, you could use some of the practical ideas suggested in this chapter to draw up your timetable.

_____

_____

_____

_____

_____

_____

_____

_____

_____

_____

_____

_____

_____

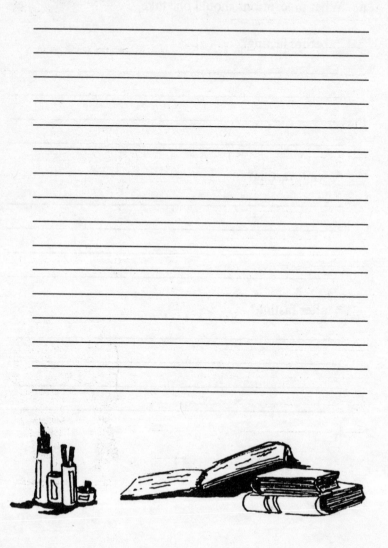

Reflection

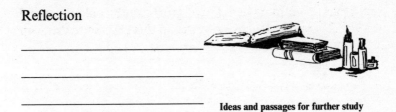

_____

_____

_____

Ideas and passages for further study

Prayer

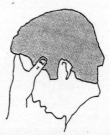

_____

_____

_____

_____

_____

**Ideas for strengthening and deepening my
prayer-life**

Action

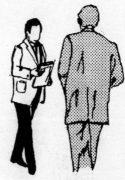

_____

_____

_____

_____

_____

Ideas to put into practice

131

CHAPTER 5   FASTING AND HEALTH

1. What is fasting, from a medical standpoint?

2. How does one feel while fasting?

3. What happens during a prolonged fast?

4. Longer or shorter fasting

5. Terminating a fast and starting to eat again

6. Who should avoid fasting?

Any fool can fast, but it takes wisdom to begin and end a fast correctly.

George Bernard Shaw

For this chapter, the author has called upon the specialized knowledge of doctors who have studied this question. Occasionally reference is made to a doctoral thesis presented to the Faculty of Medicine at Marseilles, France.

1. What is fasting, from a medical standpoint?

When a person fasts, he or she abstains from food. However the body needs food in order to live. Food provides saccharides, lipids and proteins, all of which are necessary for life to continue. Without these essential nutrients, the body is bound to die sooner or later – despite the existence of sophisticated chemical mechanisms for adapting to unusual conditions like fasting.

A person can fast in different ways: the body is accustomed to going without food at night. A brief fast lasts less than a week. A prolonged fast can last for several weeks – as in famine conditions or during hunger strikes.

The essential saccharides, lipids and proteins, mentioned above, all of which are obtained from our daily meals, are metabolized in the body to produce sugar (glucose), amino acids and fats. In the following explanation, one nutrient is more important than all the others. It is glucose. All the different tissues of the body need to take in glucose daily. However, certain tissues need it particularly and use it as their main source of energy. They are the red and white blood cells, the kidneys, the intestine, the retina, the muscles – during exercise – and especially the nervous system. During a prolonged fast with its accompanying risks, the nervous system makes use of other substances instead of glucose, using the hydrocarbons stored in the fatty tissues.

How does fasting affect the body's metabolism?

Fasting for a shorter or longer period provokes very different metabolic responses. During the early days of fasting, the body tissues, and especially the brain tissues, no longer receive their supply of sugar. Faced with this new situation, the body has to adapt in order to provide glucose to those tissues that depend on it. To do so, it draws on small quantities of glucose stored in the liver to produce 'fresh' glucose in the liver; it also uses proteins present in the muscles, which leads to them being weakened and, if pursued indefinitely, could lead to death. The longer the fast, the slower calories are burned. As fasting continues, because of the depletion of the stock of stored glucose in the liver, more hydrocarbons in the fatty tissues are metabolized to produce glucose. As a result, the concentration of uric acid – the substance responsible for gout when too great a quantity is present in the blood – increases.

The liver is not the only organ in which glucose is stored. The kidneys too share in its production; and they serve to eliminate the ammonia produced as waste product during metabolism of proteins present in the muscles.

After fasting for about three days, one observes an increase in the ammonia present in one's urine. This indicates a reduced elimination of urea, the normal waste product of metabolism, which tends to reduce the need for water. In this way, to some degree, human beings are able to adapt to a temporary fast by drawing from the reserves of energy stored in the liver, in the muscles and in the fatty tissues. This enables them to spend energy continuously, though eating only intermittently – under normal conditions, three times a day.

During a period of eating normally, the 'fuel' taken in more than covers the immediate need for energy, so much of it is stocked for future use.

During a period of fasting, the body draws from its reserves of energy. The nervous system and hormonal mechanisms regulate these modifications of the body's metabolism.

Fasting does temporarily affect the whole digestive system: the taste buds, normally stimulated by eating, begin to atrophy; the salivary glands begin to dry up, and the secretions produced by the mucous membranes begin to decrease in quantity and quality, and even to disappear.

Drinking water (the source of life) helps the body to tolerate fasting better by slowing down the inevitable process of dehydration. Remember that water constitutes a major part of most foods and composes 60% of the body's weight.

Any individual is able to fast, involuntarily or voluntarily. However, sooner or later, and depending on their physical condition, fasting will produce the previously mentioned changes in the body's metabolism, resulting in a real decrease in their physical and intellectual performance.

Some individuals and some races tolerate a short fast better than others. This is due to the fact that the needs of the body vary according to climate and to a person's sex, weight, age, usual physical activities and eating habits (the amount eaten, the kind of food, the number of meals per day). Other variables include differing performance from one individual to another based on inherited genetic characteristics.

In affluent western society, marked by all kinds of excesses, undernourishment is rare. The undernourishment so common in developing countries is, in reality, a kind of enforced, artificial fast.

Though one can speak about a 'balanced meal', it is quite wrong to speak of 'balanced fasting'.[18]

2. How does one feel while fasting?

'One needs to be aware that the first forty-eight hours are not always easy and pleasant. Headaches, stomach burns, nausea and giddiness may occur. However, these unpleasant sensations disappear gradually, and in the end completely. They are simply an expression of the body's desire for its usual nourishment. Nonetheless they are somewhat similar to the pain felt by someone who is suddenly deprived of stimulants like tea, coffee, alcohol, tobacco, spices and seasoning: the process of elimination is somewhat painful, but its effects are beneficial.'[19]

'Our appetite for food (wrongly called hunger) makes itself felt in the stomach. This kind of "hunger" is simply due to habit and in no way implies that food is really needed. One simply wants to fill one's stomach in order to stop the unpleasantness caused by fasting and the accompanying processes of elimination of toxins and mucus. This false sensation of hunger is very keen if the person has made inadequate preparation for fasting. Nonetheless, subsequently it disappears completely.

'Real hunger generally occurs only when one starts eating again. Like real thirst, it is felt in the mouth and throat.'[20]

The benefits of fasting

After fasting for one or two days, most people feel lighter, more comfortable and relaxed. In fact, they are surprised to feel so well.

– 'Fasting allows the body to recuperate its run-down stock of energy since, physiologically, it is a period of rest.

– 'Fasting accelerates and intensifies the elimination of toxins.

– 'By obliging the body to depend on its own internal resources, fasting provokes the rapid suppression – by a process called autolysis – of growths, infiltrations, deposits, accumulations, superfluous or pathological tissues.

'These are examined by the body in detail and their useful constituents are employed to nourish the vital tissues, while their useless ones are excreted.

– 'Fasting allows the body to regenerate itself by the previously mentioned processes associated with a process of reconstruction. Physiologically, the body is rejuvenated, its functioning is improved, its structures are repaired and its vitality increased.'[21]

3. What happens during a prolonged fast?
(more than 24 hours)

'**Sight.** Sometimes one notices that one's sight decreases somewhat: one begins to confuse certain letters. However, there is no need for anxiety, one's sight soon returns to normal and sometimes even improves. However, drivers of vehicles should take care as their reflexes and concentration may be diminished.

'**Intelligence.** One may be surprised to read a chapter twice without really understanding it. One's comprehension seems to be hindered. Once again, this is no cause for anxiety, for in a few days it too will return to normal.

'**Memory.** One may find that one cannot remember as often as usual what has just been said. One may forget one's appointments or even one's own telephone number. One may have difficulty in finding one's words. This is not surprising as, for once, one's brain is also having a rest. It is a sign that, after being intellectually overworked, it is disconnecting itself.'[22]

'**Skin.** While fasting one observes a spectacular rejuvenation of one's skin: its colour becomes lighter and its texture finer.'[23]

'**Sexual capacity.** It may be modified temporarily, being either increased or decreased. After fasting, it will be improved and stabilized.

'**Periods.** They may be retarded and more or less profuse. Again, they will return to normal after terminating the fast.[24]

'**Urine.** At the beginning of a prolonged fast, urine becomes dark in colour and is accompanied by an unpleasant odour – a sign that toxins are being eliminated effectively. As the fast continues, the colour becomes light again and the odour disappears.

'**The tongue.** Like bad breath, a coated tongue is a sign of effective elimination during the early days of a prolonged fast. It may remain coated throughout the fast, but in general it gradually regains its usual colour long before starting to eat again.[25]

It is very important to observe the rules of good hygiene while fasting. Make sure that your breath is not unpleasant for those with whom you live!

'**Sleep.** Half of those who undertake a prolonged fast sleep less well and wake up more often than usual. In such cases, it is wise to avoid taking part in animated discussions, undertaking intense intellectual work or watching violent programmes on television. A short walk before going to bed will prove very beneficial. In winter, one should turn down the heating and air the bedroom well.

'**Tiredness and weakness.** During one's fast, one may suddenly feel exhausted, but this sensation disappears after a little rest. For this reason it is wise not to fast during working hours.

'**Chilliness.** One may also have a sensation of cold in one's feet or hands or even all over one's body. This is due to a slowing up of the blood circulation. One should be careful about draughts; if necessary one should wear warm clothing, have hot drinks and use a hot-water-bottle in bed.

'**Emotions.** Fasting makes one more sensitive and emotional. The longer the fast, the more the blood is purified and the more fluid it becomes, resulting in clearer and more lucid thought. While fasting, one is very sensitive to other people. Their attitudes or words can encourage or hurt. One is also more sensitive to right and wrong.'[26]

4. Longer or shorter fasting

It is possible to fast for a short period – like missing a meal or two – while continuing one's daily work. However, it is preferable and wiser to plan a more prolonged fast – lasting three or fours days – during one's holidays or over a long weekend. If in doubt, consult your doctor.

5. Terminating a fast and starting to eat again

The famous writer, George Bernard Shaw, who was familiar with the practice of fasting, observed: 'Any fool can fast, but it takes wisdom to terminate a fast correctly.'[27]

Why is terminating a fast so complicated?

It is a question of returning to normal eating and so of setting in motion again the body's usual digestive functions and metabolism.

The change from fasting to eating is slower than the change from eating to fasting. While fasting, the body interrupts its production of digestive juices. This production can only be restarted gradually.

Before starting a fast, it is necessary to learn how to terminate a fast – how to break-fast!

In fact, medically speaking, the way one starts eating again is an essential part of the fast. It requires as much time, care and attention as fasting itself.

To avoid trouble and to allow the production of digestive juices to begin again normally, one must especially observe four main rules:

- Return gradually to normal eating.

- Eat slowly: avoid swallowing hastily.

- Chew thoroughly: this is where the digestive process starts.

- Eat balanced meals: meat, vegetables, fruit, milk products . . .

6. Who should avoid fasting?

* Those who have doubts about the practice of fasting.

* People whose profession demands concentration and good reflexes: they should avoid fasting during working hours.

* Mentally ill patients with diminished capacities.

* Overworked people who are suffering from physical and nervous exhaustion. Instead they need a time of rest.

* People who have lost weight as a result of illness or of following a severe diet.

* Children.

* Diabetics and heart patients.

* Expectant mothers.

* People under medical treatment.

* People with medical concerns about their health – because their blood pressure is either too high or too low, or because they suffer from some chronic illness – should never fast without first consulting their doctor.

Reflection

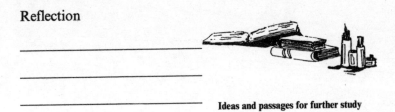

Ideas and passages for further study

_____

Prayer

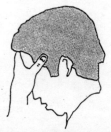

Ideas for strengthening and deepening my prayer-life

Action

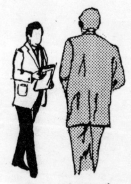

Ideas to put into practice

CONCLUSION

The aim of this book is not to encourage you to become expert at fasting, but simply to direct your attention to the biblical passages dealing with fasting and to allow you to draw your own conclusions. Before reading what follows, why not take a pencil and a sheet of paper and summarize in one or two sentences the gist of the biblical teaching on fasting? If that proves too difficult, read again Isaiah 58:1–14 and Matthew 6:1–24 where this teaching is summed up.

Is God for or against the practice of fasting?

God is *against* fasting when it is practised with a legalistic attitude, or out of a slavish respect for tradition, or as a result of a negative attitude to the body, or in order to attract attention to oneself, or to exert pressure on God himself.

God is *against* fasting when there is a sharp contradiction between appearances and reality, in other words between the act of fasting and the accompanying attitude of heart: 'Although they fast, I will not listen to their cry' (Jer. 14:12).

God is *for* fasting when it is undertaken to please him, and in a spirit of humility and of dependence, and when it is accompanied by feeding on his Word: 'Is not this the kind of fasting I have chosen . . . ?' (Isa. 58:6).

'But as for me, it is good to be near God' (Ps. 73:28). From time to time it is good for me to leave aside my projects, my appointments, my preparation for preaching, my visits, my correspondence, and occasionally one or two meals – in order to be completely 'available for God'.

APPENDIX 1.

FASTING IN THE HISTORY OF THE CHURCH

1. The intertestamental period

2. The beginnings of Christianity

3. Fasting in the fourth and fifth centuries

4. The Eastern church

5. The Reformers

6. Preachers and revivalists

A good knowledge of history helps us to understand our own times and live our lives more wisely.

Herbert Luethy

We will not repeat here what we have learned about the practice of fasting in the Bible, but will concern ourselves first of all with the period between the Old Testament and the New Testament.

1. The intertestamental period

'During the intertestamental period and even later, fasting became ever more important in Jewish piety. As a result Gentiles considered fasting as one of the distinctive marks of the Jews.

'Suetonius, the Roman historian, reports a brief extract from a letter written by Augustus to Tiberius in which he claims to have fasted as rigorously as the Jews would have done on the sabbath!' (In fact, the Jews do not fast on Saturdays but they called every day of the week a sabbath.)[28]

2. The beginnings of Christianity

'In contrast to the sobriety of the New Testament, the early Christians of the first to fifth centuries exaggerated the benefits of fasting. From the second century onwards, fasting was clearly considered as a meritorious, sacrifical work.

'Both the Western and the Eastern branches of the church have inherited the theology of the first five centuries of Christianity. As a result their conception of fasting has been deeply influenced by post-biblical writings.

'Since Jesus did not make any laws about fasting and since customs varied from one place to another, the need was gradually felt to establish rules in order to harmonize the practice of the church.

'Regular fasting appeared in the second century. Fasting before Easter was made obligatory for all the faithful. According to the place, it could last one or two days or even six.'[29]

'The church recommended fasting and saw it as a work of charity with a view to sharing with those in need. This idea would become a favourite with the church Fathers: fasting with a view to giving.

'In his "Fifth Similitude" written in the second century, Hermas advised abstaining from all but bread and water, then calculating the cost of a real meal and giving the amount to a widow, an orphan or a poor person.'[30]

a. The Didache

The Didache is an anonymous work dating from the first century. It supplies precious information about the organization of the early churches, their liturgy and the attitude of the faithful towards ministers of the gospel. Its fifteen chapters deal with subjects like baptism, the Lord's Supper and the return of Christ. It encourages the practice of fasting on Wednesdays and Fridays – not the same day as the Pharisees.

Chapter 7 recommends that candidates for baptism and those baptizing them practise fasting before entering the waters of baptism:

'Concerning baptism, baptize in this way. Having first rehearsed all these things, "baptize in the name of the Father and of the Son and of the Holy Spirit" (Mt. 28:19), in running water. But if running water is not available, baptize in other water, and if cold water is not available, then in warm. If you have neither, pour water on the candidate's head three times "in the name of the Father and of the Son and of the Holy Spirit". Before the baptism, let the baptizer and the baptized fast, and others too if they can. At least instruct the baptized to fast one or two days beforehand.'[31]

The Didache also mentions fasting before Easter: 'Beginning on Monday, during the days leading up to Easter, this obligatory fast permits the absorption of bread, salt and water; but on Friday and Saturday, fasting must be complete: nothing may be eaten.' (Canon 22)

b. Tertullian and Origen

Tertullian (160–215), jurist and theologian, defended the practice of fasting.

Born at Carthage in the middle of the second century, Tertullian was converted about the age of forty. He brought to the service of his new faith all the fire of his passionate nature. The first Christian author to write in Latin, he rendered great service to the church in creating theological terms like Trinity, sacrament, etc.

Tertullian reacted violently and fought strongly against the clericalism and latitudinarianism (free-and-easy attitude) prevalent in the institutional church of his day.

Tertullian became a convert to Montanism. The Montanists rejected the authority of the church in favour of the authority of the Holy Spirit who had spoken through the Scriptures and who still spoke through prophetic men (and women) like Montanus, who was born in Asia Minor.

Tertullian wrote a treatise on fasting and addressed it to the 'psychic' (carnal) Christians, i.e. those belonging to the 'great church' (the institutional church). This treatise is the oldest work devoted wholly to the subject of fasting, written by a Christian writer. It is at once a defence of Montanist practices and a bitter satire on fasting as practised in the 'great church'.

At that time, considerable freedom reigned in the church: there were few obligatory fasts. On the other hand, the Montanists considered the 'stations' (sacred places for prayer) to be obligatory every Wednesday and Friday. In addition, for two weeks each year, except on Saturdays and Sundays, they abstained from food such as meat, sweet fruit, wine, etc. and ate only bread and dried fruit. This practice of eating only dry food (called '*xerophagy*') was rejected by the 'great church'.

The arguments in favour of fasting drawn from the Scriptures by Tertullian were subsequently repeated by many later writers.

Origen (185–254) was the father of biblical interpretation and systematic theology.

He was born into a Christian family in Egypt. His father, Leonidas, was arrested in 202, at a time of savage persecution during the reign of Septimius. Origen wanted to die with his father, but was prevented from doing so by his mother. At the age of eighteen, when persecution was rife, he was called upon to succeed Clement of Alexandria as head of the catechetical school.

Origen lived abstemiously, slept sparingly and worked tire-lessly. A gifted orator, he also wrote commentaries on every book of the Bible and presented the whole of Christian doctrine in a systematic manner.

Note this quotation from one of his writings on prayer:

'Prayer is not so much a petition as participation in the life of God.'

Here is what he says about fasting:

'We must not fast in accordance with Jewish law, but in the spirit of the gospel. Fasting is not to be a superstitious observance but a virtuous abstinence.'[32]

'Blessed is he who fasts in order to feed the poor.'

'Origen also uses the term fasting as a metaphor for longing for the return of Christ in glory and of purifying oneself in the hope of his appearing.'[33]

3. Fasting in the fourth and fifth centuries

On account of the persecution that was rife during the reign of Decius, *Antony* (251–356) sought complete solitude in the Egyptian desert. He retired from the world in order to pray, to fast and to battle against the flesh and evil spirits. Hermits like Antony sold all their possessions, lived alone and inflicted severe austerity on themselves in the attempt to resist tempta-tion. In Antony's view, fasting constituted a way back to Paradise.

Simeon the Stylite (390–459) was a famous anchorite. For 20 years he lived in a monastery in Syria. Then he built a pillar 60 feet high, topped by a platform, and lived on it for 37 years. Perched on his platform, he preached and counselled. Thousands of people came long distances in order to listen to him and to consult him. When he died, a monastery was built on the site of his pillar.

Simeon is said to have abstained from both food and water for forty days. As a result of his going to such extremes, others began to advise moderation:

'We do not impose fasting in extreme ways or depriving oneself of food too severely, for weak bodies break down and become sick . . . One should not fast to the point of having palpitations or of scarcely being able to breathe . . . but only in order to crush the desires of the body.'[34]

It was at this period that Lent was instituted.

a. Lent

Lent, a fast preceding the festival of Easter, is mentioned for the first time in a canon of the Council of Nicea in AD 325.

It was a complete fast, lasting originally for one or two days, then for a week, and finally for forty days.

It was based on the symbolic significance of the number forty, associated in the Bible with a period preceding the establishing of a covenant between God and his people. At the time of the Flood, rain fell for a period of forty days; later, Moses and Elijah fasted for forty days before God revealed himself to them; Jesus himself fasted for forty days in the desert; in addition, the people of Israel wandered in the desert for forty years before entering the Promised Land.

The Latin word for Lent – *quadragesima* – means 'fortieth', since it began on the fortieth day before Easter, called Ash Wednesday (which falls at the end of February or in early March).

'It is a question of abstaining from meat on Fridays and of fasting on Ash Wednesday and on Easter Friday and Saturday.'[35]

Initially a complete fast compulsory for all, Lent gradually became a partial fast (missing one meal a day), with children, elderly people and sick people being exempt.

In Catholic thought, Lent has always had three meanings:

Lent is seen as an expression of repentance and conversion

As we saw previously, the early church instituted a fast in order to prepare the new converts ('*catechumens*') for the ceremony of baptism which took place in the context of the liturgy for Easter. Lent was a prolongation of this fast.

'When the church no longer baptized adults and when the institution of the catechumenate no longer existed, the basic significance of Lent remained: offering oneself to God in order to implore his mercy and forgiveness; renewing one's conversion with the acute sensation of being exiled far from God. This theme explains why, during the patristic period, the liturgy made frequent use during Lent of the parable of the prodigal son.'[36]

Lent is seen as a commemoration of Christ's forty days of fasting in the desert and of his conflict with the tempter.

The church Fathers and the liturgical tradition saw in Christ's fasting in the desert a counterpart to the temptation of Adam in the garden and a remedy for the Fall.

Lent is seen as a way of sharing in the cross of Christ and in his sufferings.

'Christ's fast was seen as an acted parable of his whole redeeming work, and our participation in his fast as a mystical sharing in his work of redemption.'[37]

b. Quarterly fasting

'Like Lent, these fasts were a late institution. The goal of these quarterly fasts was to solemnize the four seasons. There was also the additional thought of the fasts in the 4th, 7th and 10th months mentioned in the Bible.'[38]

Quarterly fasting was obligatory and involved abstinence from food for three days during the first week of each of the four seasons. It was abolished by the Second Vatican Council.

c. Eucharistic fasting

Before taking the sacrament of communion, the priest and the congregation had to fast from midnight of the previous day. This fast was reduced in 1953 to three hours, and in 1956 to one hour.

d. Monastic fasting

Pachomius (287–346), an Egyptian, was the first to have the idea of gathering several monks under the same roof. The first monastery was founded in 320, at the abandoned village of Tabennisi, on an island situated on the river Nile.

Living in community was intended to help the monks practise holiness.

'The traditional teaching of the western church sees fasting as a source of unity and cohesion for the whole Christian community. In western monasticism, fasting is practised in a rigorous way. It is intended to make us conscious of our solidarity with all Christians and with all mankind: "We are creatures of the same God and sons of the same Father," declared Pope Leo III (who died in 816 and was canonized in 1673), "so that both justice and charity demand that we deprive ourselves for the benefit of our under-nourished brothers, experiencing at least occasionally their poverty and destitution. By sharing their condition, we show brotherly love to our neighbour" (Sermon 11.1).

'Thus fasting, which for monks was primarily a way of putting their individual lives in order, now became a way of re-establishing a certain parity in society.

'In the best tradition of the early centuries of the church, fasting is not only a way of reinforcing prayer but also a way of, to some degree, giving one's life for one's neighbour.'[39]

4. The Eastern church

'Ancient eastern monasticism practised fasting in a very rigorous way. From its earliest days, eastern monasticism included fasting in its ascetic programme. On the one hand, fasting helped one combat evil spirits successfully; on the other, it allowed the spirit to meet God.'[40]

In the Eastern church, fasting is a way in which the soul devotes itself completely to preparing to celebrate worthily the various religious festivals, and especially Christ's passion. It is accompanied by religious instruction and prayer. The Eastern theologians attribute great benefits to fasting: they consider it a way to assist human weakness, to resist evil and to live with God, it enables one to pray, it is a source of wisdom and it brings peace. Thus it is the greatest of all blessings!

5. The Reformers

The Reformers were not opposed to fasting, but they strove to remove its abuses and to restore its original character.

Martin Luther (1483–1546)

Luther was in favour of celebrating a fast together in preparation for the great Christian festivals: Christmas, Easter, Whitsun and Friday evening each week. On the other hand, he was opposed to fixing an official day of fasting. He thought that, in reality, the best way to fast was to keep one's body in subjection at all times.

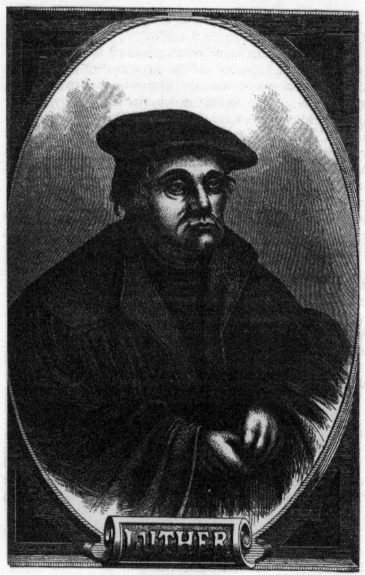

Martin LUTHER

Luther dealt with the subject of fasting in his *Treatise on Good Works* (1520). In his consideration of the Ten Commandments, Luther interpreted the third Commandment (concerning the sabbath rest) as a spiritual duty involving giving oneself inward rest and leisure by mortifying one's sinful desires. Fasting is the first 'physical exercise' contributing to this inner rest. Fasting must be regulated in the light of this spiritual goal – rather than by observing external rules relating to frequency and duration, to abstinence from one kind of food or another, or to the observance of a particular day. No authority, such as a religious order or the church itself, can determine the degree of fasting that is necessary and sufficient; each individual must decide in accordance with his own needs and convictions.

In dealing with 'good works', which include not only fasting but prayer, almsgiving, pilgrimages, building churches and celebrating festivals, Luther proclaimed: 'All of these have value only if accompanied by faith; in themselves, such works have no value for (contrary to what many imagine) they have no merit in themselves.'

John Calvin (1509–1564)

Calvin dealt with fasting in his *Institutes of the Christian Religion*.

He identifies three purposes: To 'mastering the flesh' (of which Luther spoke), he added 'preparing us for prayer' and 'expressing our humility before God'.

His main concern was to make fasting spiritually profitable. This required the correction of several mistakes: hypocritically emphasizing the outward act; erroneously considering fasting as a meritorious work performed in

God's service; dictatorially imposing fasting and making it more important than anything else – as was the case in a certain religious tradition. In his view, Lent was not justified by the Gospels: in fasting, Christ did not set us an example to follow.[41]

'Fasting, whether public or private, is an outward sign of inward sorrow. It is neither meritorious nor worthy of any praise.

'In joining fasting to prayer as an aid and a reinforcement, [Christ] indicated that it is useless by itself.

'We need to understand the right use of fasting to avoid falling into superstition.'[42]

The first national synod of the French reformed churches held at Paris expressed the same point of view as Calvin. The attitude of the Reformation is well expressed in Article 26 of the Confession of Augsburg:

'We teach that each must exercise his body by fasting . . . in order not to give way to sin, but not claim to merit grace by these works. Moreover, this discipline is not to be limited to certain days but to be continual.'

In times of persecution, the Protestant churches often celebrated days of fasting proclaimed by their synods. Even today certain churches observe an annual day of fasting, however it is usually only a day of repentance and humiliation.

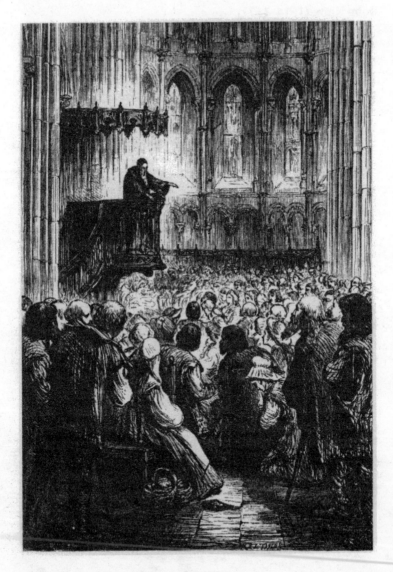

Calvin preaching his last sermon

John Knox (1514–1572)

The first Scottish Protestants were persecuted. One of them, John Knox, spent nineteen months as a galley slave in France. After being released, he stayed at Geneva on several occasions and became an enthusiastic disciple of Calvin. After returning to his native Scotland, he converted many of the nobility to the Protestant cause. His preaching stirred thousands as he thundered against idolatry and immorality.

At one point he fasted and prayed until the Lord removed Mary Stuart (the persecutor of the Protestants) from the throne, sending her first into exile in England and later to the gallows. The history books recount how she feared the prayers of John Knox more than all the armies of Queen Elizabeth I.

Knox practised fasting to a remarkable degree. Many leaders of the Reformation in England – among whom figured Latimer, Ridley and Cranmer – were martyred as a result of their strong convictions and their unshakeable faithfulness to the Word of God. Like Knox, they too not only prayed constantly but fasted regularly.

The Genevan fast

Following the massacre of thousands of Huguenots throughout France that took place in 1572 on the night of August 23–24 – the eve of Saint Bartholomew's Day – the Genevan authorities proclaimed a day of fasting, repentance and humiliation.

In his book, *Livre de Blaise*, Philippe Monnier recounts how this fast was instituted:

'On Monday, 1st September, the ministers of the Word of God asked to be heard by the Council. Gravely but calmly, they entered the town hall. They did not cry out for vengeance. They lifted neither their voices nor their fists to curse and insult. They were not troubled by doubts. They proclaimed that the doctrine they taught was sure and certain. They even insisted that if God were pleased to give Geneva the honour of suffering in a similar way for his name, this would be cause to praise and glorify him. They encouraged the city councillors to be of good courage and declared it would be wise to forestall the wrath of God by an exceptional time of prayer and fasting.

Their request was granted and a fast was celebrated on Wednesday 3 September 1572, both before and after the special time of prayer held at 3 o'clock.

Thus Geneva responded to the insult launched against its faith and law by an act of contrition, of humility and repentance.'

Even today this fast continues to be celebrated on the second Thursday of September in Geneva Cathedral.

The Church of England

After the Reformation, the Anglican church retained Lent and some other fasts practised by the Catholic church. However none of them were made obligatory. Indeed, fasting before the communion service does not figure in the official list of fasts drawn up by the Church of England, although the faithful were encouraged to prepare for taking communion by prayer and fasting. The Revised Prayer Book, presented to parliament in 1928, includes the following statement which reveals certain aspirations:

'Receiving the Holy Sacrament after fasting is an ancient and praiseworthy custom of the Church. However, to avoid confusion, we declare hereby that such preparation is not obligatory, each person being free to decide conscientiously before God whether or not to fast.'

6. Preachers and revivalists

John Wesley 1703–1791 (founder of the Methodist churches)

'John Wesley taught and practised fasting. He sought to restore the teaching and recommendations of the Didache which encouraged fasting twice a week. The first Methodists faithfully followed his example and practised fasting on Wednesdays and Fridays. Fasting was an essential part of their personal and community piety.

He protested against two extreme positions concerning fasting: "Some experience religious fasting to a degree that goes well beyond both Scripture and reason, while others have completely given up fasting." '[43]

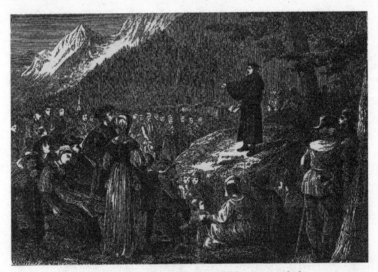

A great open-air meeting during the 18th century revival

In 1756, the king of England proclaimed a day of prayer and fasting at a time when it was feared that the French were about to invade England. In his Journal, John Wesley recounts how 'that day the churches were full and the prayers were fervent. It was a glorious day. God heard our prayers and this contributed to the maintenance of peace and tranquillity in our country.'

George Whitefield (1717–1770)

A contemporary of John Wesley, George Whitefield was the champion of vast meetings in the open-air. For thirty-four years, thousands thronged to hear him preach the gospel. He too often practised prayer and fasting.

We could also cite the examples of Jonathan Edwards (1637–1716) and of Charles Finney (1792–1875), of Pastor Hsi of China and of Hudson Taylor (1832–1905), the famous missionary to China who often practised fasting.

In the United States, several fast days with a view to public prayer and humiliation were proclaimed during the 18th and 19th centuries.

Charles Haddon Spurgeon (1834-1892)

Called 'the Prince of Preachers', Charles Spurgeon preached to 6000 people every Sunday. During his 38-year-ministry of preaching and teaching at the Metropolitan Tabernacle in London, he saw 14,692 people added to the church. He often proclaimed days of prayer and fasting. This is how he described those days:

'Our days of fasting and prayer were a great blessing to us all. The gates of heaven were wide open and our hearts tasted the glory of God.'

However, in general, fasting was not widely practised in the churches descended from the Reformation. When believers fasted, it was usually individually and privately. The examples of group fasting mentioned above were rather exceptional.

In the Catholic church, the practice of fasting has gradually declined through the centuries. By the twentieth century, ascetic fasting had become little more than a distant memory.

Personal Notes

APPENDIX 2

FASTING IN THE MAJOR WORLD RELIGIONS

1. Primitive religions

2. Judaism

3. Islam

4. Hinduism

5. Buddhism

1. Primitive religions

'In the primitive religions, fasting was practised on the occasion of the New Year festival, an agrarian festival celebrated with a view to regenerating cosmic forces. In the course of these festivals celebrating the New Year, the expulsion of the old year was accompanied by that of all the evils and sins committed by the people as it ran its course.

Fasting was almost always associated with rites of renewal, of initiation and of mourning. It was seen as a kind of transfer of energy to the mysterious powers that made nature fertile. The simplest and most effective means to prevent these powers from becoming troubled, weakened or angry was to strengthen them with food. The way to feed them was by depriving oneself of food: one abstained from food in order to preserve the power present in the food from being contaminated as a result of contact with one's own impurity. Conversely, by fasting one sought to prevent evil powers present in one's food from gaining entry into oneself.

These are not the only meanings of fasting in primitive cultures where the practice is always accompanied by a wider set of restrictions concerning behaviour in the areas of work, speech, expressions of joy and sexual activities, all intended to create a climate of sadness and affliction.'[44]

2. Judaism

Fasting on the occasion of religious festivals

For the Jews, a festival is a time set aside for worship and holy celebration. Fasting is recommended and practised for many of these festivals.

The festivals recalled great events in Jewish history and various encounters between God and his people. The most important are mentioned in the Torah (the first five books of the Old Testament).

Rosh Hashana

The Torah mentions 'days of austerity'. The Jewish New Year lasts two days. On this anniversary of the creation of the world and of the sacrifice of Isaac by Abraham, the Jew implores God to write his name in the Book of Life. It is also seen as the annual opening session of the Divine Tribunal. After examining people's conduct, God decides (as the liturgy puts it) 'who will live and who will die, who will experience happiness and who will experience tribulation . . .' 'But . . . prayer, repentance and charity can diminish the severity of the divine verdict.' Hence the fervent prayers at this time, underlined by the sounding of a ram's horn (the *shofar*), which recalls the ram sacrificed by Abraham instead of Isaac after God has rescinded his instruction to put him to death.

The following ten days are a period of penitence leading up to 'the great Day of Pardon' (Yom Kippur, the tenth day of the seventh month, *Tisri* = September–October), anniversary of the day on which God forgave his people their sin in worshipping the golden calf.

Yom Kippur

On the Day of Atonement (Lev 23:26–32), the people fast and pray for twenty-four hours in the synagogue. Kippur has become the most important of all the Jewish religious festivals: not only do even the least practising flock to the synagogues, but religious services are also held on other premises specially prepared for the occasion.

'From sunset to the appearing of the stars the following day, the people fast completely and pray continually, confessing their faults to God. They recite an exhaustive catalogue of all possible sins using the first person plural. In this way they express the solidarity of all the people with the sins committed by each of them. Thus, it is hoped, the purity of the innocent will attenuate the guilt of the sinners and obtain their forgiveness. The power of repentance to obtain remission is recalled by the public reading of the book of Jonah. The service ends with the sevenfold repetition of the proclamation of God's oneness: "The Lord alone is God!" quoted from the story of the prophet Elijah on mount Carmel.'[45]

In chapter 8 of his book entitled *Yomah*, a famous rabbi called Judah the Saint (135–217 A.D.) recounts the practical details of how the Day of Atonement was celebrated in his day. Many more prohibitions are mentioned than in the book of Leviticus:

'On the Day of Atonement, it is forbidden to eat or drink, to wash or anoint the body, to wear shoes or to have marital relations . . .' (*Yomah*, 8:1).

However, life itself is more important than Kippur, so neither children (*Yomah*, 8:3) nor expectant mothers nor the sick (*Yomah*, 8:4) are compelled to fast.[46]

Note also the importance and meaning of this festival for Philo of Alexandria, a Greek philosopher of Jewish origin born in 13 BC Philo presents the Day of Atonement as the most sacred of all festivals:

'This day is doubly significant: it is at one and the same time a day of rejoicing and also a day of purification and deliverance from sins.

This festival teaches self-discipline since it is entirely devoted to supplication and intercession. It comes just after harvest-time. Abstaining from starting immediately to eat the produce harvested is an act of piety by which one recognizes that it is God who is able to feed one and keep one alive.'[47]

Purim (a Persian word for *fate* or *lot*)

'This Jewish festival was instituted between 486 and 465 BC in order to commemorate the deliverance of the Jewish exiles during the reign of king Xerxes. When Haman, his prime minister, plotted to exterminate them, God used Esther and her tutor Mordecai (both of them Jews themselves) to save his people (Est 8:20–28).

Right from the start, the feast of Purim proved very popular. It has always been observed at the same date. On the 13th day of *Adar* (February), the Jews fast; in the evening (the beginning of the 14th), they meet in the synagogues. The service begins with the reading of the book of Esther. When the name of Haman is read, all shout: "Wipe out his name!" or "The name of the wicked will vanish". The young people especially make a great noise as they repeat all the names of Haman's sons in one breath – in order to recall the fact that they were all hung together. The following morning, everyone comes back to the synagogue and concludes the festive ritual before going out to celebrate. The rich distribute gifts to the poor."[48]

The anniversary of the destruction of the Temple

In the year AD 70, the Jerusalem Temple was destroyed on the 9th day of the month of *Ab* (July–August). Ever since, the Jews have fasted on this day as a sign of mourning.

Despite the difficulties posed by their dispersion and the numerous attempts made to exterminate them, the ritual of fasting has continued to be passed down from father to son. The Jews fast before Rosh Hashana, for Yom Kippur, to prepare for Purim, and in memory of the Temple. Fasting is an integral part of the thought, prayer and life of the Jewish people. In their view, fasting serves a triple purpose: to expiate sin, to purify the sinner in the eyes of God, and to enable the rich to share with the poor.

During the period between the Old and New Testaments and even afterwards, fasting became more and more important in Jewish piety, to such an extent that non-Jews considered it one of the distinctive marks of the Jewish people.

Prayer, almsgiving and fasting are three essential pillars of Jewish piety.

'Judah the Saint, a rabbi who lived during the second century A.D., called a council with a view to recording in writing Jewish jurisprudence – the opinions of the most important teachers on the interpretation of the Law. The book thus composed was called "*the Mishnah*", which means "the repetition of the Law".'[49]

The *Mishnah* deals with fasting several times, particularly in the books of *Ta anit* and *Yomah*.

The first three chapters of *Ta anit* refers to occasions on which fasting should be appointed: for example, when rain is withheld and drought occurs, and in times of disaster due to plagues, locust invasions or floods.

3. Islam

Muhammad

According to Muhammad, prayer takes us halfway along the path that leads to God and fasting brings us to the gates of heaven.

One who for forty days engages in the purest form of prayer (viz. abstaining from food and drink) – is said to know 'the joy of sensing the springs of wisdom rise from his heart to his lips'.

Before starting out on his mission, Muhammad himself practised fasting in the underground caves found in the region of Mecca. While fasting in the course of these solitary retreats, he had several mystical experiences of a prophetic nature. It was during his fast at Hira, in the month of Ramadan, that the Koran is said to have been revealed to him.

The place of fasting in the Koran

The ninth lunar month, called Ramadan, was chosen because it was the month in which Muhammad, the prophet of Islam, received his revelations: 'The month of Ramadan is that during which the Koran was revealed in order to show men the right path with all desirable exactness and to enable them to distinguish between good and evil. Whoever among you sees the new moon must fast during this whole month . . .' (Sura 2:183–185).

The rules laid down by the Koran are as follows: 'Eat and drink until you can distinguish at dawn between a white thread and a black thread, then fast strictly until nightfall' (Sura 2:187).

Fasting and pilgrimages

Muslims who go on a pilgrimage to Mecca are obliged to fast for three days on the outward journey and for seven days on the return journey.

Each year, in the month of *I-hijja*, pilgrims flock to the Great Mosque and perform a 'circumambulation' around the sanctuary (*Kaaba*). This rite is practised with much zeal by a vast number of people.

Fasting while on a pilgrimage is intended to compensate for those unable to offer an animal as a sacrifice: 'For the love of God, undertake the pilgrimage to Mecca . . . According to your means, you should offer an animal as a sacrifice. He who does not possess an animal must fast for three days at the time of pilgrimage instead of offering a sheep, and for seven days when back home, making ten whole days in all . . . Whatever good you do, God will know about it.' (Sura 2:196–203).[50]

The Ramadan

Muslims throughout the world have an appointment once a year with the moon, or rather with the crescent-shaped new moon which marks the beginning of the month of Ramadan. It corresponds to the ninth month of the Muslim religious calendar.

Prayer and fasting are obligatory throughout the whole of the month for all Muslims.

The Ramadan is a major obligation for every devout Muslim. Indeed, it is one of the 'Five Pillars' (foundations) of Islam. The others are: the recital of the brief Muslim creed (professing faith in one God); the obligation to pray five times a day at stated hours; almsgiving (the amount of which is fixed by law); and the performance of at least one pilgrimage to Mecca.

For a whole month, from dawn to dusk (i.e. from about 6 am to about 6 pm), it is forbidden to eat or drink or smoke, and to engage in sexual intercourse or to entertain impure thoughts. However, children, pregnant women and nursing mothers, sick people and travellers are all exempt from fasting.

When the sun sets on the horizon, fasting is interrupted amidst great, and sometimes noisy, rejoicing – hence the term '*randam*', meaning 'din'. People sit up all night until dawn, eating and reciting chapter after chapter of the Koran.

For the Muslim, fasting itself constitutes a way of praying physically: one's mind and body must be concentrated wholly on meditation, God and one's neighbour. Considered an act of courage requiring great self-discipline, fasting is seen as a way of making amends for one's faults and of obtaining the forgiveness of God. In addition, it is said to contract the conduits of the body through which sin is thought to circulate. Muhammad claimed that fasting, accompanied by prayer, was the only way to secure relief from oneself.

4. Hinduism

In Hinduism too, ascetic practices (including fasting) are considered to be a means of liberation. This idea is based on the theory that inaction is superior to action. Inaction means first of all, abstaining from killing, and then abstention from any kind of action.

Fasting is an integral part of Hinduism. Hindu literature mentions fasting constantly, and even today millions of Hindus fast at the slightest pretext. Fasting is considered an essential part of prayer, and the mortification of the body's desires is thought to be indispensable to spiritual progress.

The history of Hinduism is marked by a number of people who fasted to an exceptional degree. Perhaps the best-known is Mahatma Gandhi (1869–1948).

Gandhi

'An Indian philosopher, Gandhi strove for the independence of India. He based his action on the principle of non-violence. After studying as a young man in London, he began his career as a lawyer in South Africa. He returned to India in 1917 and became involved in the movement to win national independence.

'At first Gandhi's fasts were motivated by his respect for Hindu tradition, by his childhood memories, and by his concern to link mental health with physical health. Despite being attracted by the teachings of the Bible and of the Qur'an, Gandhi remained firmly rooted in Hinduism. He used to fast during several days in memory of his parents who had been devout Hindus. He remembered that his mother, Putlibai Gandhi, was accustomed to observe both those fasts in honour of the goddess Shiva and also the one-night fast (*prashe*) traditionally observed during the fifth month of the year (*sravan*).

'At thirty-seven years of age, Gandhi took up fasting on the first and eleventh days of the lunar month. These fasts were compulsory for worshippers of the god Vishnu who would spend the night reading their sacred writings. To these obligatory fasts, Putlibai Gandhi added voluntary ones.

'Like all orthodox Hindus, Gandhi was a vegetarian. He soon became very concerned about the influence of food on people's behaviour. Devoted to the principle of non-violence (*ahimsa*), he attributed great importance to the strict observance of an exclusively vegetarian diet, accompanied by meticulous attention to the quality and quantity of food involved.

'For Gandhi, fasting was also a "spiritual means" to unite
different religions. He longed to reconcile Hindus, Muslims
and Christians. He thought it essential for fasting to be a
sincere expression of one's personal faith.He also opposed
fasting in a spectacular way, for he thought that playing religious games of this sort would prove suicidal to both Hinduism
and Islam. Aspiring to forge a new unity between Hindus and
Muslims, he saw fasting as having both spiritual and political
significance for both populations.

'In 1907, the *sravan* fast (in the fifth month of the Hindu
year) coincided with the Muslim fast of the Ramadan. At the
Tolstoy farm that he created and ran with the help of his friend
Kallenbach, Gandhi encouraged the four or five Muslims who
lived on the farm to observe the Ramadan and invited the local
Hindus, Parsees and Christians to join them in its observance.

'Gandhi considered fasting a kind of voluntary death or
self-sacrifice. "I don't fast for my own pleasure," he confessed.
"Nor do I torture my body in order to become famous.
However, I endure with joy the pangs of hunger and other
unpleasant sensations associated with fasting – from which no
one will imagine that I am exempt. These fasts are only
endurable because they are imposed on me by a higher power
and also because this power gives me the ability to endure the
suffering entailed."

'Gandhi always insisted that fasting requires great purity
and is accompanied by suffering. "The purer the suffering,"
he wrote, "the greater the spiritual progress."

'For Gandhi, fasting was a way by which the mind could gain
mastery over the body. He himself declared: "Fasting undertaken in order to attain the most perfect self-expression and
in order that the mind may become master of the body, is one

of the most powerful factors of our spiritual progress." "Fasting is an essential part of my life. I could no more do without it than I could do without my eyes. Indeed, just as my eyes enable me to see the external world, so fasting gives me insight into the inner world."

'On several occasions, Gandhi used fasting as a weapon for non-violent combat. He went on hunger-strikes in order to fight against injustice by exerting pressure on various governments in the hope of overturning their projects. In this way he was determined to combat the "impurity" of the whole of humanity.

'In January 1932, on returning to India from a conference held in London, he was arrested and jailed. In August of that year, while still in prison at Yeravda, he learned that the British government intended to create separate electoral colleges in the various parliaments for the Untouchables. As the apostle of unity both between religions and within Hinduism itself, he could not accept what he saw as a form of "vivisection". When a government minister named MacDonald confirmed this decision on 17th August, Gandhi announced that, unless the government rescinded its decision, on the 20th September he would begin fasting and continue until he died. He held out against all opposition, rejecting all pleas to accept a compromise, and pursued his fast until finally the government gave in to his demands.'[51]

5. Buddhism

'Buddhism owes its origin to a certain Siddharta Gautama, son of a North Indian prince who lived during the 6th and 5th centuries BC. The name Buddha is actually a title meaning "The Enlightened One".

'Buddhist doctrine can be summed up in what are called "the Four Noble Truths":

- Suffering is universal.

- The cause of all the suffering in the world is desire.

- The only way to escape suffering is to quench desire.

- The only way to quench desire is to follow "the Noble Eightfold Path".[52]

Buddha

In order to obtain the release of his spirit from matter, Buddha had imposed long periods of fasting on himself. Following a period of forty days and forty nights spent solely in fasting and meditation while seated under a lime tree, he believed he had discovered the answer to his questions concerning the origin and destiny of humanity and the laws of the universe.

'While mortifying the body in typically ascetic fashion some years before his "Awakening", he reduced his intake of food to such an extent that he nearly died. However, after realising that traditional ascetic mortification was of no value, he had begun once again to eat the normal and sufficient quantity of food. After his "Awakening", he advised his disciples that if eating too much is one extreme, eating too little is another.

'Buddha's disciples ate and slept little. Copious meals and the deep sleep they induce were obstacles on the road to renunciation since they made it impossible to meditate, to be vigilant and to make spiritual progress. In order to practise effective contemplation and prolonged meditation, it was necessary to limit one's intake of food. However the sacred texts did not specify the precise amount of food prescribed for a monk.

'A Buddhist monk was permitted to eat only one meal a day: "If a monk eats solid food outside of the right time (i.e. between sunrise and midday), he commits a fault belonging to the category '*Pâittiya*' (Commentary on the Vinaya, 4:85)." '[53]

A monk was allowed to eat meat only if the animal had been killed for him by someone else. He lived on alms and accepted the food people gave him. He was forbidden to express a desire for a particular kind of food.

The monk's meal was accompanied by a specific meditation:

'First of all, what am I worth? Where has this offering come from? Secondly, if I accept this food, I must think hard about my weakness of character in doing so. Thirdly, I must keep a watch over my heart in order to avoid faults such as excessive desire etc. (this is the most important) . . . Fourthly, I must take this food like good medicine – simply to preserve the health of my body. Fifthly, I must accept this food with a view to making progress spiritually.'

'The first mouthful is with a view to renouncing all evil, the second with a view to doing all manner of good, the third with a view to saving all sentient beings so that each can finally attain the state of Buddha (the Enlightened One).'[54]

Today, some Buddhists still practise fasting with a view to purifying themselves spiritually.

Fasting is practised by Buddhists especially in Tibet where Buddhism is combined with the pre-Buddhist religion of Tibet called shamanism.

NOTES

Chapter 1

1. Martinez, P., *Psychologie de la Prière* (Valence, L.L.B. 1990) p. 32.
2. Peyrous, D.R., *La Spiritualité* (Paris, Que Sais-Je, P.U.F., 1988) p 83.
3. Martinez, P, op. cit., p. 32.
4. *La Bible Annotée*, Vol. 4 (St Légier, Ed. Emmaüs).

Chapter 2

5. Lemaître, D. and E., *Le sens du jeûne* (Nouan-le-Fuzelier, Ed. Pneumathèque, 1993) p. 52.
6. Ibid. p 45.
7. Carson, D.A., *Teach Us To Pray* (Carlisle, Paternoster 1994).
8. Foster, Richard, *Celebration of Discipline* – Revised Edition (London, Hodder and Stoughton, 1989).
9. Dumas, André, *Cent Prières Possibles* (Ed. Cana, 1982) p. 154.
10. Gotte, Catherine, *Pour une meilleure compréhension du jeûne dans la piété chrétienne* (Thesis presented to the Free Faculty of Evangelical Theology, Vaux-sur-Seine, Maison-Alfort, 1981)
11. Foster, op. cit.
12. Carrel, Alexis, *L'homme, cet inconnu* (Paris, Ed. Plon, 1935)

Chapter 3

13. Used by permission of Mr P. Guesche of the North Africa Gospel Mission.
14. Martinez P., *Théologie de la prière* (Valence, L.L.B., 1995) p. 46.
15. Carson, D.A., op. cit.

Chapter 4

16. Martinez P., op. cit., p. 50.
17. Saury, Alain, *La régénération par le jeûne* (St Jean de Braye, Ed. Dangles, 1978)

Chapter 5

18. Perraut, Dr A. *Le jeûne et la prière*, article in brochure no. 35 of S.I.P. Voyages, p. 11 (May 1985), used by permission of Mme Chantal Flocard, editor of the publication *"Itinéraires chrétiens"*.
19. Ray, Maurice, *Pour que nous soyons libérés*, Théologie Pratique Vol. 4 (Lausanne, LLB, Ed. Emmaüs 1986), p. 132.
20. Saury, op. cit., p. 146
21. Lebrun, Corinne, *Un traitement naturel: le jeûne* (Doctoral thesis presented to the Faculty of Medicine of Marseilles, 1989) p. 71.
22. Lutzner, Dr H. *Comment Revivre par le jeûne* (Ed. Terre Vivante, Paris 1984)
23. Lebrun, op. cit.

24. Lutzner, op. cit.
25. Saury, op. cit.
26. Saury, ibid., p. 147.
27. Lutzner, op. cit., p. 64.

Appendix 1

28. Thomassin Lovis, *Traité des jeûnes de l'Eglise* (Ed. Louis Roulland, 1693), p. 11.
29. Moreau E. *Jeûne et abstinence aux premiers siècles de l'Eglise*, (Nouvelle revue théologique, Vol 61, 1934), p. 743.
30. Lemaître, op. cit.
31. Nicole, J.M. *Précis de l'histoire de l'Eglise* (Ed. Institut Biblique de Nogent-sur-Marne, 1994) p. 20.
32. Origen, *Homelies on Leviticus* (Feuillet) 10.
33. Ibid., 269.
34. Jerome, *Letters*, 130, 11
35. Grousset, Véronique, *Guide pratique du Catholicisme* (Ed. First, 1995) p. 159.
36. Placide, Deseille, Jeûne, article in *Dictionnaire de la spiritualité* (Paris, G. Beauschesne et Cie, 1974) p. 1170 and 1171.
37. Vogüé, Adalbert de, *Aimer le jeûne* (Ed. Cerf, 1988) p. 39.
38. Gagnon E.M., *Le jeûne et la prière* (S.I.P. Voyages, May 1985).
39. Ibid.
40. Vogüé, ibid, p. 101.
41. Calvin, John, *Institutes of the Christian Religion*, a new translation by Henry Beveridge, London, Clarke, 1957) Book 4, 12:20.
42. Ibid.
43. Foster, op. cit.

Appendix 2

44. Deseille, op. cit., Vol 8, p. 1165.
45. Coirault, M., *Les fêtes juives, chrétienne, musulmanes* (Paris, Ed. Cerf).
46. Quotations from *Yomah* are taken from the Jerusalem Talmud, Vol. 5, pp. 247–257.
47. Philo of Alexandria, *De Specialibus Legibus Liber*, Vol. 1: pp. 121, 187, 193–198).
48. Coirault, op. cit.
49. *Introduction, Jerusalem Talmud*, translation M. Schwab (Maurice Liber, Paris, Librairie orientale et américaine, 1932) Vol. 1, pp. xii, xiii.
50. Lebrun, Corinne. 'Un traitement naturel: Le jeûne' (doctoral thesis, Marseilles) pp. 29, 30.
51. Drevet, Camille, *La Redécouverte du jeûne* (Paris, Ed. du Cerf).
52. Nicole, J.M., *Précis d'histoire des religions* (Ed. Institut Biblique de-Nogent-sur-Marne, 1990) pp. 124, 126.
53. Wijayaratna, Mohan, *Le moine bouddhiste selon les textes du Theravâda* (Paris, Ed. du Cerf)
54. Suzuki D.T., *Essais sur le bouddhisme zen* (Spiritualités vivantes) p. 383.

BIBLIOGRAPHY

(References to works quoted or consulted)

1. Reference works in French

La Bible annotée, Vol 4 (O.T. Kings to Esther), edited by F. Godet. P.E.R.L.E. (St-Légier, Switzerland, Ed. Emmaus).

Dictionnaire de la spiritualité, edited by Jacob-Kyspenning, (Paris, G. Beauchesne et Cie, 1974).

Dictionnaire de théologie (Paris, Ed. Cerf, 1988).

Nouveau Dictionnaire Biblique (St Légier, Ed. Emmaüs, 1992)

La redécouverte du jeûne (Paris, Ed. Cerf, 1991).

Vocabulaire de théologie biblique (Paris, Ed. Cerf, 1991)

2. Titles in French

Cohen A.	*Le Talmud* (Ed. Payot).
Coirault M.	*Les fêtes juives, chrétiennes, musulmanes* (Paris, Ed. Cerf).
Darricau & Peyrous	*La Spiritualité* (Paris, Que sais-je? P.U.F.1988)
Drevet C.	*La Rédécouverte du jeûne* (Paris, Ed. Cerf).
Dumas A.	*Cent prières possible* (Condé-sur-Noireau, Ed.Cana, 1982).
Eastman D.	*L'heure qui change le monde* (Deerfield, Ed. Vida).
Flory R.D.	*Le jeûne biblique et la prière* (booklet) 1973.
Gibson O.J.	*En avant n° 1*, (Pierrelatte, Ed. Biblos, 1979)
Gotte C.	*Pour une meilleure compréhension du jeûne dans la piété chrétienne* (thesis presented to the Free Faculty of Evangelical Theology, Vaux-sur-Seine, Maison-Alfort, 1981).
Grousset V.	*Guide pratique du Catholicisme* (Paris, Ed.First, 1995).
Gugenheim E.	*Le Judaïsme dans la vie quotidienne* (Ed. Albin Michel, 1978).
Lebrun C.	*Un traitement naturel: le jeûne* (Doctoral thesis presented to the Faculty of Medicine of Marseilles, 1989).

Lemaître D & E — *Le sens du jeûne* (Nouan-le-Fuzelier, Ed. Pneumathèque, 1993).

Lützner H. — *Comment revivre par le jeûne* (Paris, Ed.Terre Vivante, 1984)

Martinez P. — *Pratique de la prière* (Valence, Ed. LLB, 1996).

Martinez P. — *Psychologie de la prière* (Valence, Ed. LLB, 1996).

Martinez P. — *Théologie de la prière* (Valence, Ed. LLB, 1990)

Moreau E. — *Jeûne et abstinence aux premiers siècles de l'Eglise* (Nouvelle revue théologique; Vol. 61, 1934).

Newberry Y. — *Le désir et le plaisir de prier* (Pierrelatte, Ed. Biblos, 1987)

Newberry Y. — *La prière, j'y crois* (Pierrelatte, Ed. Biblos, 1993)

Newberry Y. — *Un retour à l'essentiel: Dieu* (Pierrelatte, Ed. Association Séminaires, 1986)

Newberry Y. — *Au coeur de la prière* (Pierrelatte, Ed. Biblos, 1992).

Nicole J.M. — *Précis d'histoire de l'Eglise* (Ed. Institut Biblique de Nogent-sur-Marne, 1994).

Ray M. — *Pour que nous soyons libérés* (Lausanne, Ed. LLB, 1986).

Saury A. — *La régénération par le jeûne* (St Jean de Braye, Ed. Dangles, 1978).

Sourdel D.	*L'Islam,*(Paris, Que-Sais-Je? P.U.F., 1949)
Thomassin L.	*Traité des jeûnes de l'Eglise*, (Ed. L. Roulland, 1693).
Vogüé A. de	*Aimer le jeûne* (Paris, ed. Cerf, 1988)
Weiss E.	*Choul'hâne Aroukh abrégé*, (Paris, Ed. Fondation Sefer, 1980).
Wijayaratna M.	*Le moine bouddhiste selon les texte du Theravâda* (Paris, Ed. Cerf).

3. Titles in English

Behm J.	Fasting, article in *Kittel's Theological Dictionary of the NT* (1942) Vol. 4.
Brown C. (Ed.)	*Dictionary of New Testament Theology* (Exeter, Paternoster, 1975)
Calvin J.	*Institutes of the Christian Religion*, (London, Clarke, 1957)
Carson D.A.	*Teach Us to Pray* (Carlisle, Paternoster, 1994)
Douglas J.D.	*The New International Dictionary of the Christian Church* (Exeter, Paternoster, 1974)
Duewel W.	*Touch The World Through Prayer* (Bromley, S.T.L., 1987)
Elwell W.A. (Ed.)	*Evangelical Dictionary of Theology* (Grand Rapids, Bakers 1984).

Forster R.T.   Fasting, article in *New Dictionary of Christian Ethics and Pastoral Theology*, (Leicester, IVP, 1995).

Foster R.   *Celebration of Discipline*, Revised Edition (London, Hodders, 1993).

Harris, Archer &Waltke   Article in *Theological Wordbook of the Old Testament*. (Grand Rapids, Zondervan).

Johnstone P.   *Operation World* (WEC International, 1993).

Lewis J.P.   Fasting, article in *The Zondervan Encyclopedia of the Bible* (Grand Rapids, 1975-76), Vol. 2, pp. 501–4.

Lloyd-Jones D.M.   *Studies in the Sermon on the Mount*, Vol. 1 (London, IVP, 1960) pp. 33–44.

Packer J.I.   *Knowing God* (London, Hodder and Stoughton, 1973).

Scroggie W.G.   *How To Pray* (Grand Rapids, Kregel, 1955)

Shallis R.   *From Now On* (Carlisle, S.T.L., 1987)

VanGemeren (Ed.) Article in *The New Theological Dictionary of the OT* (Carlisle, Paternoster, 1997)

Wallis A.   *God's Chosen Fast* (Eastbourne, Kingsway Publications, 1987)

Index

S

T

V

W

Y

Z

A PERSONAL CONTACT WITH THE AUTHOR

I invite you to write me a few lines giving me your remarks, criticisms and encouragements. I would like you to do so in order to establish a contact between us, to enable us to pray one for another, and to improve the contents of this book with a view to a future edition. If you wish, you could simply copy and answer the following questions:

1. How did you obtain this book?

2. Were you able to read all the chapters?

3. Which chapter helped you the most and why?

4. Are there any aspects of fasting which are not mentioned in the book and which ought to be included in a future edition?

5. Have you any other suggestions for improving the book?

6. Have you been able to use any of the ideas mentioned in the book in your prayer group or church? Which ones?

7. Is there anything else you would like to share with me?

Would you kindly reply to –

Ian Newberry,
Editions Biblos,
628, Avenue Teilhard de Chardin
26700 Pierrelatte France

Other books by Ian Newberry

Back To Basics : Back To God   Price £6.00

At The Heart of Prayer   Price £6.00

Enjoying God's Presence   Price £1.00

Kindly send your order to :   Seminars on Prayer
Back to Basics
c/o Iain Smith,
36 Berelands Crescent,
Rutherglen,
GLASGOW,
G73 1XW
Scotland.

Please wait until you receive your bill before sending your payment as we will include the package costs in your bill. Thank you.

If you are interested about the possibility of organizing a seminar on prayer in your church, please write to:

Mr Iain Smith, Prayer Seminar Co-ordinator, at the above address.

BACK TO BASICS

BACK TO GOD

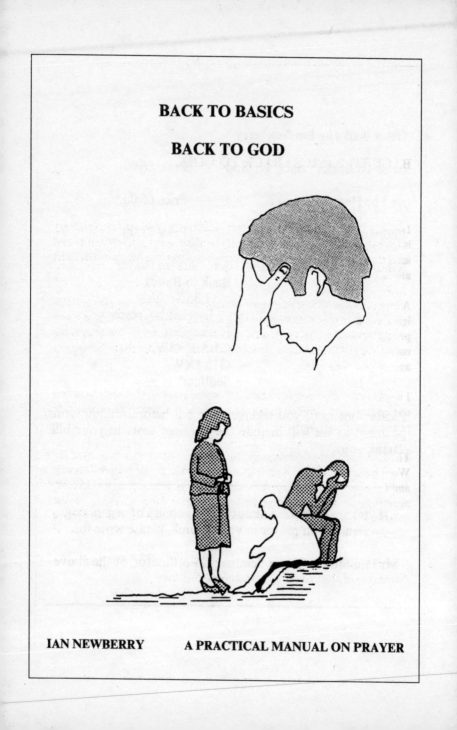

IAN NEWBERRY   **A PRACTICAL MANUAL ON PRAYER**

BACK TO BASICS : BACK TO GOD

I am excited about the prayer seminars that my close friend Ian Newberry is organising. I believe that the prayer life of the average Christian as well as of the Church in general is one of the most important things on the heart and mind of God.

A lot of us seem to misunderstand what the Bible says about prayer. This ignorance, coupled with disobedience and the extreme busyness of many people, leads the Church into the sin of prayerlessness. This affects the entire work of God in the individual and in the Church across the country and around the world.

I would really urge people to take advantage of the opportunity to attend one of these seminars on prayer, to study and put what they hear into practice on a daily basis.

The Epistle of James reminds us that we must not be only hearers of the Word but also doers. Prayer is the key to revival in our personal, family and Church life. Some have false ideas about prayer, others are discouraged because their favourite prayer has never been answered. These questions will be dealt with from the Word of God in this important seminar.

George VERWER,
International Director of Operation Mobilisation

AT THE HEART

OF PRAYER

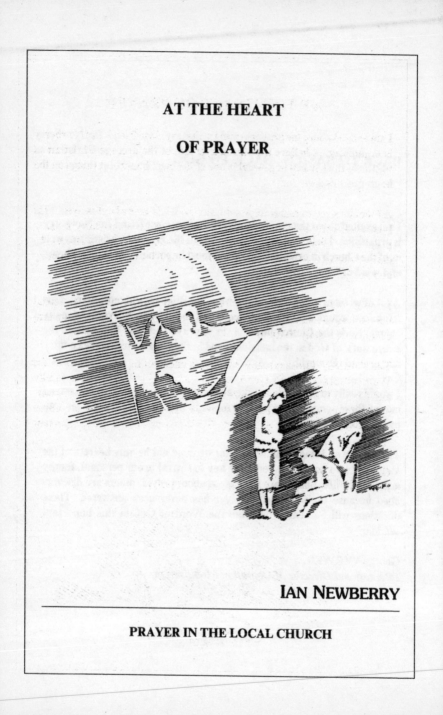

IAN NEWBERRY

PRAYER IN THE LOCAL CHURCH

AT THE HEART OF PRAYER

I am excited about the prayer seminars that my close friend, Ian Newberry is organising. I believe that the prayer-life of the average Christian as well as of the Church in general is one of the most important things on the heart and mind of God.

A lot of us seem to misunderstand what the Bible says about prayer. This ignorance, coupled with disobedience and the extreme busyness of many people, leads the Church into the sin of prayerlessness. This affects the entire work of God in the individual and in the Church across the country and around the world.

I would really urge people to take advantage of the opportunity to attend one of these seminars on prayer, to study and put what they hear into practice on a daily basis.

The Epistle of James reminds us that we must not be only hearers of the Word but also doers. Prayer is the key to revival in our personal, family and Church life. Some have false ideas about prayer, others are discouraged because their favourite prayer has never been answered. These questions will be dealt with from the Word of God in this important seminar.

George VERWER,
International Director of Operation Mobilisation

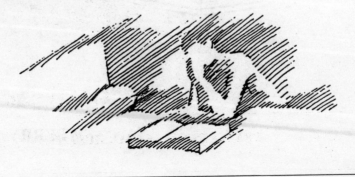

ENJOYING

GOD'S PRESENCE

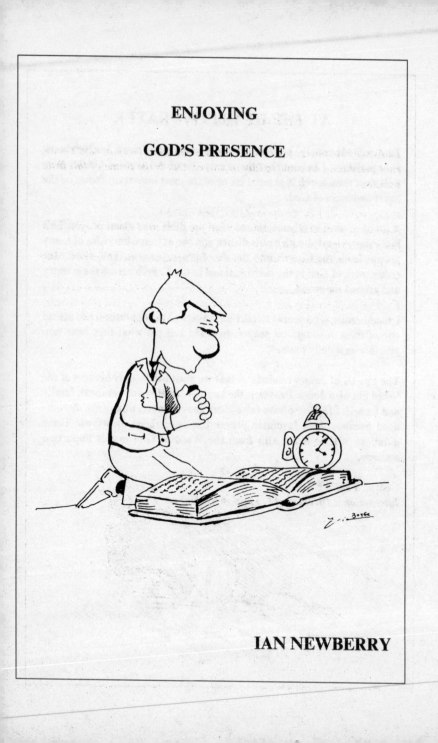

IAN NEWBERRY

Enjoying God's Presence

Rediscovering peace, joy, intimacy and the thrill of being in God's presence every time we come to him in prayer, that is the theme of this little booklet.

A new method? No. An up-to-date approach? No.
Another sentimental gimmick that will get us excited about prayer for a few days, then fizzle out? No.
Another legalistic law to reinforce our guilt complex about prayer? No.

To rediscover and cultivate a fresh spontaneous joy in God's presence, this booklet suggests that our prayers be rooted in God – a God who is here, who is alive, who is powerful and who wants us to enjoy his presence.

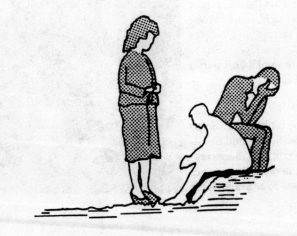

AVAILABLE FOR GOD
Ian Newberry

Fasting has been taught and practised in the major world religions like Hinduism, Buddhism and Islam, and by great religious leaders like Confucius, Zoroaster, Gandhi and the Indian yogis. It was mentioned by great philosophers like Plato, Socrates and Aristotle and also by Hippocrates, the Greek physician commonly regarded as the father of medicine.

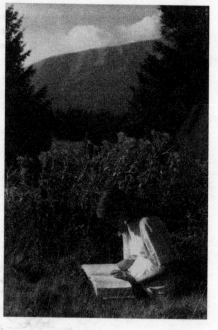

What does the Bible teach about fasting? What does Jesus say?

For what purpose, in what circumstances and in what way can we fast personally? What about collective fasting? What are the differences between right and wrong ways of fasting?

What are the biblical norms for fasting?

This book invites you to discover the biblical answers to these questions – and to discover that fasting means **taking time to enjoy the presence of God and to be available for God.**